MRCP 1
Clinical Sciences

Best of Five Questions and Answers

Geraint Rees MRCP, PhD
Wellcome Senior Clinical Fellow in Biomedical Science,
University College London, UK and
Honorary Consultant Neurologist,
National Hospital for Neurology and Neurosurgery.

Egerton Court
Parkgate Estate
Knutsford
Cheshire
WA16 8DX

Telephone: 01565 752000

First Published 2006
ISBN: 1 90462734 X

A catalogue record for this book is available from the British Library.

Text prepared by Carnegie Publishing, Lancaster
Printed and bound in the UK by MPG Books Ltd

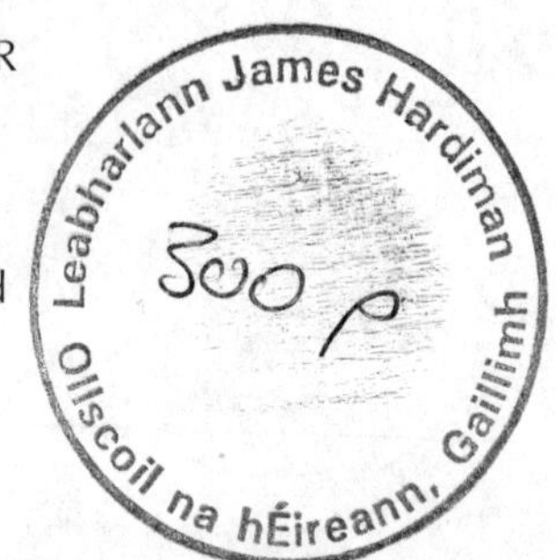

CONTENTS

Correct answers and teaching notes follow the questions in each chapter.

FOREWORD

Clinical science is the most important topic in the MRCP (UK) Part I exam, currently accounting for 25 of the 200 questions across the two papers. These 25 questions are broken down by the Royal College of Physicians into the following topic areas:

Cell, molecular and membrane biology	2
Clinical anatomy	3
Clinical biochemistry and metabolism	4
Clinical physiology	4
Genetics	3
Immunology	4
Statistics, epidemiology and evidence-based medicine	5

This book presents 300 original 'best of five' clinical science questions. Unlike previous MCQ publications, the questions are divided exactly in proportion and topic according to the Royal College of Physicians distribution given above. I hope that this will give candidates a good idea of the range and proportion of clinical science questions that are likely to face them in the MRCP examination, together with pointers to appropriate learning material. Many questions are accompanied by a brief explanation, and uniquely cross-referenced further to brief revision note summaries of each topic that are contained in the companion volume *Essential Revision Notes for MRCP*, 2nd edition by P A Kalra, which is also published by PasTest.

Geraint Rees MRCP, PhD
London, January 2006

Chapter 1

CELL, MOLECULAR AND MEMBRANE BIOLOGY

Questions

---

1. Which one of the following hormones uses cAMP (cyclic adenosine monophosphate) as its intracellular messenger?

- ☐ A ACTH (adrenocorticotrophic hormone)
- ☐ B TRH (thyrotrophin-releasing hormone)
- ☐ C Insulin
- ☐ D GnRH (gonadotrophin-releasing hormone)
- ☐ E GH (growth hormone)

2. What is the most likely mode of action of aspirin?

- ☐ A Cyclo-oxygenase pathway
- ☐ B ADP receptor blocking
- ☐ C Glycoprotein GPIIb/IIIa activity
- ☐ D Platelet modulation
- ☐ E cAMP synthesis

Answers on pages 11–18

3. What is the most likely function of the protein P53?

- ☐ A Cell membrane receptor
- ☐ B Tumour promoter
- ☐ C Hormone
- ☐ D Second messenger
- ☐ E Cell cycle regulation

4. What is the most common function of nitric oxide (NO)?

- ☐ A Neurotransmitter
- ☐ B Inotrope
- ☐ C Vasodilator
- ☐ D Chronotrope
- ☐ E Vasoconstrictor

5. Which one of the following is associated with the mechanism of action of insulin?

- ☐ A Hormonal receptor DNA binding
- ☐ B Tyrosine kinase activity
- ☐ C G-protein-coupled receptor
- ☐ D Ligand-gated ion channel
- ☐ E Stimulation of hepatic gluconeogenesis

6. In which one of the following diseases is there most likely to be detectable circulating levels of interleukin-1β (IL-1β)?

- ☐ A Creutzfeldt–Jakob disease
- ☐ B Acute rheumatoid arthritis
- ☐ C Primary biliary cirrhosis
- ☐ D Hypertension
- ☐ E Acute renal failure

7. Which one of the following is a nuclear hormone?

- ☐ A Vitamin K
- ☐ B Vitamin D
- ☐ C Vitamin C
- ☐ D Vitamin E
- ☐ E Vitamin B_{12}

8. Which one of the following phenomena is associated with apoptosis?

- ☐ A S phase of the cell cycle
- ☐ B Cell lysis
- ☐ C Necrotic cell death
- ☐ D Programmed cell death
- ☐ E Free radical toxicity

Answers on pages 11–18

9. The pathogenesis of which one of the following infections results from abnormal G-protein function?

- ☐ A Cholera
- ☐ B Rabies
- ☐ C Herpes simplex encephalitis
- ☐ D Typhoid
- ☐ E Tuberculosis

10. Which one of the following hormones does not use an intracellular second messenger?

- ☐ A Insulin
- ☐ B Glucagon
- ☐ C Somatostatin
- ☐ D Epinephrine (adrenaline)
- ☐ E Insulin-like growth factor I (IGF-I)

11. What is the most likely infective agent in variant Creutzfeldt–Jakob disease (vCJD)?

- ☐ A Bacterium
- ☐ B Virus
- ☐ C DNA
- ☐ D Protein
- ☐ E RNA

12. What is the most likely general function of proto-oncogenes in normal cells?

- ☐ A DNA repair
- ☐ B Cell cycle inhibition
- ☐ C Promotion of apoptosis
- ☐ D Control of cell growth
- ☐ E Intercellular signalling

13. Which one of the following genetic disorders shows anticipation?

- ☐ A Myotonic dystrophy
- ☐ B Klinefelter syndrome
- ☐ C Down syndrome
- ☐ D Marfan syndrome
- ☐ E Duchenne dystrophy

14. Into which one of the following cell types are monocytes most likely to differentiate?

- ☐ A Red blood cells
- ☐ B Mast cells
- ☐ C Kupffer cells
- ☐ D Langerhans' cells
- ☐ E Glial cells

Answers on pages 11–18

15. Which one of the following is an intracellular protein that is most likely to be upregulated after DNA damage?

- ☐ A ICAM-1 (intercellular adhesion molecule-1)
- ☐ B Ras
- ☐ C Endothelin-1
- ☐ D NO
- ☐ E P53

16. Which one of the following hormones binds to G-protein-coupled receptors on the cell surface?

- ☐ A GH
- ☐ B ACTH
- ☐ C Oestrogen
- ☐ D TSH (thyroid-stimulating hormone)
- ☐ E FSH (follicle-stimulating hormone)

17. Which one of the following is most likely to be caused by tumour necrosis factor-α (TNF-α)?

- ☐ A Increased levels of P53
- ☐ B Enhanced insulin sensitivity
- ☐ C Inhibition of IL-1 expression
- ☐ D Programmed cell death
- ☐ E Activation of the nuclear factor κB (NF-κB) transcription factor

18. Which one of the following features is characteristic of a transcription factor?

☐ A Binds DNA

☐ B Binds RNA

☐ C Located in cell nucleus

☐ D Located in endoplasmic reticulum

☐ E Protein phosphorylase activity

19. What would be the most appropriate technique to characterise the entire pattern of gene expression in breast cancer?

☐ A Southern blot

☐ B Polymerase chain reaction (PCR)

☐ C Gene array

☐ D Fluorescent *in situ* hybridisation (FISH)

☐ E Comparative genomic hybridisation (CGH)

20. What is the most likely mechanism of action for anti-sense oligonucleotides?

☐ A Non-specific DNA binding

☐ B Messenger RNA (mRNA) binding

☐ C Enhances gene transcription

☐ D Induces apoptosis

☐ E Promotes IL-1 production

Answers on pages 11–18

21. What is the most likely reason why women are very occasionally affected by Duchenne muscular dystrophy?

- ☐ A Anticipation
- ☐ B Lyonisation
- ☐ C Opsonisation
- ☐ D Incomplete penetrance
- ☐ E Mitochondrial transmission

22. What is the most likely molecular mechanism for muscular weakness in myasthenia gravis?

- ☐ A Point mutation in acetylcholine receptor gene
- ☐ B Point mutation in myosin gene
- ☐ C Antibodies to striated muscle
- ☐ D Antibodies to acetylcholine receptors
- ☐ E Antibodies to smooth muscle antibodies

23. Which molecular technique would be most appropriate for screening for the sickle-cell mutation?

- ☐ A Northern blot
- ☐ B Western blot
- ☐ C Southern blot
- ☐ D FISH
- ☐ E CGH

24. Which one of the following disorders is most likely to involve apoptosis?

- ☐ A Cystic fibrosis
- ☐ B Graft-versus-host disease (GvHD)
- ☐ C Acute transfusion reaction
- ☐ D Anaphylaxis
- ☐ E Cardiac failure

Answers on pages 11–18

CELL, MOLECULAR AND MEMBRANE BIOLOGY

Answers

1. **A: ACTH**

The conversion of extracellular signals, via intermediates or second messengers, into changes in the internal state of a cell is central to all cellular processes. Peptide and amine hormones act via cAMP (eg all pituitary hormones except GH and prolactin), via a rise in intracellular calcium (eg GnRH or TRH) or via receptor tyrosine kinases (eg insulin, GH). *See also* Question 10.

Essential Revision Notes for MRCP, 2nd edn, p 118

2. **A: Cyclo-oxygenase pathway**

Non-steroidal anti-inflammatory drugs and aspirin operate by inhibiting cyclo-oxygenase, thus reducing the production of prostaglandins and thromboxane.

Essential Revision Notes for MRCP, 2nd edn, p 325

3. **E: Cell cycle regulation**

P53 is the protein transcribed from the *p53* tumour-suppressor gene and is a transcription factor (*see* Question 18), with a primary function of downregulating the cell cycle. Mutations to the *p53* gene are the most common genetic abnormality in many tumours.

Essential Revision Notes for MRCP, 2nd edn, p 441

4. C: Vasodilator

Nitric oxide (previously known as endothelium-derived relaxant factor) is produced from L-arginine by nitric oxide synthase in several different cell types, including vascular endothelium. It is a local messenger with a very short half-life which acts by activating guanylyl cyclase (giving rise to an increase in intracellular cyclic guanosine monophosphate or cGMP). NO plays a role in modulating vascular tone through its vasodilator action, but it is also involved in cell-mediated immunity.

Essential Revision Notes for MRCP, 2nd edn, p 444

5. B: Tyrosine kinase activity

Insulin binds to a cell membrane receptor protein which then undergoes dimerisation and autophosphorylation at a tyrosine residue. This activates tyrosine kinase activity intrinsic to the receptor and results in the actions of insulin through phosphorylation of cytoplasmic proteins. Insulin does not act through a G-protein-coupled receptor or an intracellular hormonal receptor. Among its many metabolic effects, insulin inhibits hepatic gluconeogenesis.

Essential Revision Notes for MRCP, 2nd edn, p 435

6. B: Acute rheumatoid arthritis

Interleukin-1 is a molecule that is synthesised by mononuclear phagocytes that have been activated by inflammation, and acts as a central regulator of the inflammatory response. Usually it is undetectable in the circulation, but during acute inflammatory episodes (eg rheumatoid arthritis, with acute organ rejection, sepsis) it rises to measurable levels.

Essential Revision Notes for MRCP, 2nd edn, p 447

7. B: Vitamin D

Nuclear hormones bind to intracellular receptors rather than use second messenger systems to give rise to intracellular changes. The receptors then bind with DNA in the cell nucleus, controlling transcription of DNA. Nuclear hormones include corticosteroids, vitamin D, retinoic acid, oestrogen, progesterone and testosterone.

Essential Revision Notes for MRCP, 2nd edn, p 436

8. D: Programmed cell death

The process of naturally occurring cell death is regulated by the activation of a specific set of genes in response to extracellular signals. This process is known as programmed cell death, and the morphological changes accompanying it are known as apoptosis. In contrast to necrosis, apoptosis is not an inflammatory process because proteolytic enzymes and free radicals are not released as part of programmed cell death. Apoptotic mechanisms are hypothesised to be dysfunctional in many diseases, including cancer (failure of programmed cell death) and some neurodegenerative diseases (inappropriate or excess programmed cell death).

Essential Revision Notes for MRCP, 2nd edn, p 442

9. A: Cholera

G-proteins bind the guanine nucleotides GDP and GTP. They are associated with the inner surface of the cell membrane and with transmembrane receptors of hormones and other extracellular signals. The Ga_s subunit (so called because it stimulates adenylyl cyclase) is the target of the toxin secreted by *Vibrio cholerae*. Binding of the cholera toxin to this subunit causes continued production of cAMP, resulting in massive salt loss from intestinal epithelial cells; the consequent osmotic fluid shifts cause the characteristic torrential diarrhoea.

Essential Revision Notes for MRCP, 2nd edn, p 435

10. A: Insulin

The insulin receptor has intrinsic tyrosine kinase activity, which can (when activated) directly phosphorylate intracellular proteins. *See also* Question 5.

Essential Revision Notes for MRCP, 2nd edn, p 118

11. D: Protein

Variant CJD is a currently rare, rapidly progressive dementia that has been identified in younger patients. It can have a prodrome of neuropsychiatric symptoms and is likely to represent the human form of bovine spongiform encephalopathy (BSE), a prion disease of cows that crossed the species barrier into humans through ingestion of infected central nervous system tissue. The infectious agent is the prion protein.

Essential Revision Notes for MRCP, 2nd edn, p 451

12. D: Control of cell growth

Oncogenes were originally identified as genes that are carried by cancer-causing viruses. Proto-oncogenes are cellular homologues in the normal human genome which are highly evolutionarily conserved and have important roles in the control of cell growth and differentiation. Mutations in proto-oncogenes are an important cause of cancer.

Essential Revision Notes for MRCP, 2nd edn, p 440

13. A: Myotonic dystrophy

Anticipation is the tendency for a genetic disorder to become more severe and present at an earlier age in successive generations. It typically results from expansion of an unstable triplet repeat in a gene. Myotonic dystrophy is an autosomal dominant disorder that results from expansion of a CTG triplet repeat in the dystrophia myotonica protein kinase (*DMPK*) gene on chromosome 19q13.3, the exact function of which is not known.

Essential Revision Notes for MRCP, 2nd edn, p 456

14. C: Kupffer cells

Monocytes are large, circulating, phagocytic, white blood cells that represent about 3–8% of the white blood cells in circulation. They are macrophage precursors and so can differentiate into Kupffer cells, which are specialised endothelial cells that form part of the reticulendothelial system in the liver. In contrast, Langerhans' cells are endocrine cells of the pancreas, mast cells derive from bone marrow precursors expressing CD38 and glial cells from embryonic ectoderm (although note that microglia are phagocytic and derived from bone marrow myeloid precursors).

Essential Revision Notes for MRCP, 2nd edn, p 280

15. E: P53

P53 is a protein that plays a pivotal role in the cell cycle. It can induce growth arrest, apoptosis and cell senescence. In normal cells P53 is usually inactive, bound to the protein MDM-2. This prevents its action and promotes its degradation. Active P53 is induced after the effects of various cancer-causing agents such as ultraviolet radiation, oncogenes and some DNA-damaging drugs.

Essential Revision Notes for MRCP, 2nd edn, p 441

16. A: GH

Insulin, GH, prolactin, IGF-I and epidermal growth factor (EGF) receptors do not use second messengers, but instead the receptors themselves act as tyrosine kinases that can phosphorylate cellular proteins, thus modulating nuclear transcription. *See also* Question 1.

Essential Revision Notes for MRCP, 2nd edn, p 118

17. E: Activation of the NF-κB transcription factor

TNF-α and -β are two non-allelic forms of TNF, a cytokine involved in systemic inflammation and the acute phase response. It is a potent stimulator of prostaglandin production and activates monocytes and macrophages in diseased tissue. TNF-α is produced by macrophages, eosinophils and natural killer (NK) cells whereas TNF-β is made by activated T lymphocytes. The transcription factor NF-$\kappa\beta$ is implicated in the regulation of the acute phase response and is activated directly by TNF-α.

Essential Revision Notes for MRCP, 2nd edn, p 448

18. A: Binds DNA

A transcription factor is a cellular protein that binds DNA at a specific promoter or enhancer region or site, where it regulates gene transcription.

Essential Revision Notes for MRCP, 2nd edn, p 437

19. C: Gene array

PCR allows amplification of small DNA sequences, which can then be detected by a Southern blot that uses electrophoresis to separate DNA fragments, the identity of which is detected using a hybridisation probe. FISH and CGH can be used to identify the presence of mutations in specific genes. However, to examine the *entire* pattern of gene *expression*, a DNA ('gene') microarray would be most appropriate. This uses isolated DNA fragments attached to a substrate, which can then selectively hybridise with a probe made from cellular RNA. This allows the simultaneous study of the expression of many cellular genes.

Essential Revision Notes for MRCP, 2nd edn, p 429

20. B: mRNA binding

An anti-sense oligonucleotide is typically a short, artificially produced sequence that is complementary to some mRNA sequence. When anti-sense DNA or RNA is introduced into a cell, it binds to mRNA molecules with that specific sequence and inactivates them, preventing synthesis of the corresponding protein. This is an extremely specific way of inactivating cellular proteins, which is of great interest as a potential form of therapy in oncology and elsewhere.

Essential Revision Notes for MRCP, 2nd edn, p 429

21. B: Lyonisation

Lyonisation is also known as X inactivation; it refers to the process whereby only one copy of an X-chromosome is active in a cell that contains more than one X-chromosome. The selection of the active X is usually random and consequently females may phenotypically express (usually in a much weaker form) an X-linked recessive genotype.

Essential Revision Notes for MRCP, 2nd edn, pp 230, 459

22. D: Antibodies to acetylcholine receptors

Myasthenia gravis is an autoimmune disease resulting from antibodies directed at the nicotinic acetylcholine (ACh) receptor on the postsynaptic membrane of the neuromuscular junction. This leads to complement-mediated destruction of the receptors and their functional blockade. This, in turn, can give rise to fatigable weakness, most commonly presenting as ptosis, diplopia and limb weakness.

Essential Revision Notes for MRCP, 2nd edn, p 458

23. C: Southern blot

PCR allows amplification of small DNA sequences, which can then be detected by a Southern blot; this uses electrophoresis to separate DNA fragments with identity being detected using a hybridisation probe. In contrast, a northern blot detects RNA (not DNA) and a western blot detects protein.

Essential Revision Notes for MRCP, 2nd edn, p 430

24. B: Graft-versus-host disease

Apoptosis describes the morphological changes that accompany programmed cell death. This is a normal phenomenon in human development and, in contrast to necrosis, apoptosis does not induce the release of proteolytic enzymes and free radicals because it is not an inflammatory process. Some disorders, such as GvHD, are associated with excessive cell death whereas others (eg cancer, autoimmunity) are associated with a failure of programmed cell death.

Essential Revision Notes for MRCP, 2nd edn, p 442

Chapter 2

CLINICAL ANATOMY

Questions

---

1. A 68-year-old man presents with crushing central chest pain and is found to have ST elevation in leads V1–V5. Which coronary artery is most likely to have been occluded?

- ☐ A Posterior descending
- ☐ B Left circumflex
- ☐ C Coronary sinus
- ☐ D Left anterior descending
- ☐ E Right coronary

2. A 54-year-old person with diabetes presents with horizontal diplopia, worse on left gaze. The outer image disappears when the left eye is covered. Which muscle is most likely to have been affected?

- ☐ A Right medial rectus
- ☐ B Right superior oblique
- ☐ C Left medial rectus
- ☐ D Right lateral rectus
- ☐ E Left lateral rectus

Answers on pages 33–43

3. An 80-year-old presents with a left homonymous hemianopia. Which area of the brain is most likely to have been damaged?

- ☐ A Left parietal lobe
- ☐ B Right occipital lobe
- ☐ C Left occipital lobe
- ☐ D Right parietal lobe
- ☐ E Right temporal lobe

4. An 84-year-old woman presents with altered sensation in her little and ring fingers and weakness of finger abduction. Which nerve is most likely to be affected?

- ☐ A Radial nerve
- ☐ B Median nerve
- ☐ C Anterior interosseous nerve
- ☐ D Axillary nerve
- ☐ E Ulnar nerve

5. At what vertebral level is the spinal cord most likely to end?

- ☐ A T12
- ☐ B T9–10
- ☐ C S1–2
- ☐ D L2–3
- ☐ E L4–5

6. A 56-year-old man develops foot drop and disturbance of sensation over the dorsum of the foot. What nerve in the lower limb is most likely to have been damaged?

- ☐ A Sciatic nerve
- ☐ B Common peroneal nerve
- ☐ C Femoral nerve
- ☐ D Obturator nerve
- ☐ E Tibial nerve

7. A 78-year-old presents with sudden onset blindness in the right eye. Where is the most likely site for the lesion?

- ☐ A Occipital lobe
- ☐ B Optic chiasma
- ☐ C Optic tract
- ☐ D Optic radiation
- ☐ E Optic nerve

8. A 76-year-old smoker presents with acute onset of flaccid leg weakness, with impaired light touch sensation to T8, but preserved vibration and joint position sense in the lower limbs. What is the most likely diagnosis?

- ☐ A Basilar artery occlusion
- ☐ B Transverse myelitis
- ☐ C Brown–Séquard syndrome
- ☐ D Acute cord compression
- ☐ E Anterior spinal artery occlusion

Answers on pages 33–43

9. A 68-year-old man is admitted after a collapse at home with left hemiplegia and urinary incontinence. Which one of the following arteries is most likely to be affected?

- ☐ A Middle cerebral artery
- ☐ B Anterior cerebral artery
- ☐ C Posterior cerebral artery
- ☐ D Vertebral artery
- ☐ E Posterior inferior cerebellar artery

10. Which one of the following disorders is most likely to be associated with reticulonodular shadowing in the basal zone of a chest X-ray?

- ☐ A Tuberculosis
- ☐ B Sarcoidosis
- ☐ C Idiopathic pulmonary fibrosis
- ☐ D Silicosis
- ☐ E Extrinsic allergic alveolitis

11. A man presents with back pain and inability to dorsiflex his right big toe. In what area are you most likely to find loss of sensation?

- ☐ A Front of right calf
- ☐ B Dorsum of foot
- ☐ C Back of right thigh
- ☐ D Buttocks and genitalia
- ☐ E Front of right thigh

12. What clinical sign is most likely to result from a unilateral cerebellar lesion?

- ☐ A Astereognosis
- ☐ B Hemiparesis
- ☐ C Athetosis
- ☐ D Intention tremor
- ☐ E Rigidity

13. Which one of the following pancreatic cell types is most likely to secrete somatostatin?

- ☐ A α Cells
- ☐ B Langerhans' cells
- ☐ C β Cells
- ☐ D Acinar cells
- ☐ E δ Cells

14. Where is the azygos lobe seen on an anteroposterior (AP) chest X-ray?

- ☐ A Right lower zone
- ☐ B Right middle zone
- ☐ C Right upper zone
- ☐ D Left upper zone
- ☐ E Left lower zone

Answers on pages 33–43

15. What structure is likely to have been damaged if there is loss of sensation on the lateral aspect of the hand?

- ☐ A C8 nerve root
- ☐ B Lower cord of brachial plexus
- ☐ C Ulnar nerve
- ☐ D Median nerve
- ☐ E Axillary nerve

16. Involvement of which one of the following anatomical structures would be more consistent with ulcerative colitis than Crohn's disease?

- ☐ A Descending colon
- ☐ B Stomach
- ☐ C Terminal ileum
- ☐ D Rectum
- ☐ E Ileocaecal junction

17. Which one of the following is most likely to result from damage to the facial nerve at the level of the geniculate ganglion?

- ☐ A Hypoacusis
- ☐ B Weakness of the forehead muscles
- ☐ C Decreased lacrimation
- ☐ D Loss of tongue sensation
- ☐ E Pupil dilatation

18. Which one of the following is most likely to result from damage to the ulnar nerve at the elbow?

- ☐ A Loss of sweating over the hypothenar eminence
- ☐ B Inability to oppose the thumb
- ☐ C Inability to adduct the thumb
- ☐ D Inability to extend the fingers
- ☐ E Loss of sensation over the dorsum of the fourth and fifth fingers

19. A 78-year-old man dies after 7 years of progressive cognitive decline accompanied by agitation and visual hallucinations. His symptoms were dramatically worsened by small doses of haloperidol. What is the most likely abnormal anatomical finding in his brain at postmortem examination?

- ☐ A Senile plaques
- ☐ B Neurofibrillary tangles
- ☐ C Lewy bodies
- ☐ D Amyloid
- ☐ E Pick bodies

20. A 37-year-old woman suffers transient left hemiparesis while being treated for a left calf deep venous thrombosis. What abnormality of cardiac anatomy is most likely?

- ☐ A Tricuspid stenosis
- ☐ B Pulmonary stenosis
- ☐ C Ventricular septal defect
- ☐ D Aortic stenosis
- ☐ E Patent foramen ovale

Answers on pages 33–43

21. Which one of the following is most likely to cause upper lobe fibrosis?

- ☐ A Allergic bronchopulmonary aspergillosis
- ☐ B Asbestosis
- ☐ C Rheumatoid arthritis
- ☐ D Scleroderma
- ☐ E Paraquat poisoning

22. A 32-year-old presents with unilateral foot drop, difficulty walking over uneven surfaces and loss of sensation on the dorsum of the foot. What anatomical location is most likely to be affected to give rise to these symptoms?

- ☐ A Spinal cord
- ☐ B Root lesion
- ☐ C Tibial nerve
- ☐ D Common peroneal nerve
- ☐ E Deep peroneal nerve

23. Which one of the following anatomical changes are most consistent with the Wernicke–Korsakoff syndrome?

- ☐ A Atrophy of the mammillary bodies
- ☐ B Degeneration of anterior horn cells
- ☐ C Dilatation of the lateral ventricles
- ☐ D Cortical atrophy
- ☐ E Damage to the lateral geniculate nucleus

24. A 23-year-old has penetrating wounds to the forearm and difficulty adducting the thumb after a knife attack. Which structure is most likely to have been injured?

- ☐ A Median nerve
- ☐ B Musculocutaneous nerve
- ☐ C Radial nerve
- ☐ D Ulnar nerve
- ☐ E Axillary nerve

25. Which anatomical structure is most likely to be damaged in a patient with visual extinction?

- ☐ A Parietal lobe
- ☐ B Temporal lobe
- ☐ C Frontal lobe
- ☐ D Occipital lobe
- ☐ E Thalamus

26. Which anatomical portion of the nephron is damaged in acute renal failure caused by gentamicin therapy?

- ☐ A Glomerulus
- ☐ B Proximal convoluted tubule
- ☐ C Loop of Henle
- ☐ D Distal convoluted tubule
- ☐ E Collecting duct

Answers on pages 33–43

27. Which one of the following anatomical structures is most likely to be an immunologically privileged site?

- ☐ A Pancreas
- ☐ B Testicle
- ☐ C Cavernous sinus
- ☐ D Ovary
- ☐ E Pituitary

28. What is the most likely location for the lesion in a patient with a left-sided Horner syndrome associated with decreased sweating on the ipsilateral face?

- ☐ A Left common carotid
- ☐ B Left internal carotid
- ☐ C Hypothalamus
- ☐ D Central cord
- ☐ E Superior orbital fissure

29. A 32-year-old woman presents with pain on arm abduction and has a small area of tenderness lateral to the acromion. Which tendon is most likely to be affected?

- ☐ A Infraspinatus
- ☐ B Supraspinatus
- ☐ C Trapezius
- ☐ D Pectoralis minor
- ☐ E Latissimus dorsi

30. An asymptomatic 31-year-old man has a systolic murmur that is louder on inspiration and quieter during a Valsalva manoeuvre. What is the most likely anatomical cause of the murmur?

☐ A Ventricular septal defect

☐ B Aortic stenosis

☐ C Tricuspid regurgitation

☐ D Aortic regurgitation

☐ E Mitral regurgitation

31. If a patient has abnormal deviation of the uvula to the right on speaking, where is the causative lesion most likely to be located?

☐ A Midbrain

☐ B Thalamus

☐ C Pons

☐ D Medulla

☐ E Cervical cord

32. Which one of the following organs lies immediately anterior to and in direct contact with the left kidney?

☐ A Splenic flexure

☐ B Tail of pancreas

☐ C Left psoas muscle

☐ D Left suprarenal

☐ E Spleen

Answers on pages 33–43

33. A 56-year-old man is admitted with central chest pain. ECG abnormalities include an R wave in V1 with 3 mm of ST depression in V1–V3 and ST elevation in leads II, III and aVF. Which artery is likely to have been involved in this acute myocardial infarction?

- ☐ A Left main stem
- ☐ B Diagonal
- ☐ C Left anterior descending
- ☐ D First septal branch
- ☐ E Right coronary

34. A 65-year-old woman with suspected Hodgkin's disease undergoes lymph node biopsy. Which histopathological finding is most likely to suggest the worst prognosis?

- ☐ A Lymphoctye predominant
- ☐ B Nodular sclerosis type II
- ☐ C Lymphocyte depleted
- ☐ D Nodular sclerosis type I
- ☐ E Mixed cellularity

35. Which of the following disorders is most likely to be associated with aortic coarctation?

- ☐ A Marfan syndrome
- ☐ B Turner syndrome
- ☐ C Klinefelter syndrome
- ☐ D Bicuspid aortic valve
- ☐ E Edwards syndrome

36. Which one of the following anatomical locations is most likely to be critical for absorption of vitamin B_{12}?

- ☐ A Stomach
- ☐ B Duodenum
- ☐ C Ileum
- ☐ D Jejunum
- ☐ E Caecum

Answers on pages 33–43

CLINICAL ANATOMY

Answers

1. **D: Left anterior descending**

   This is the classic pattern for an occlusion of the left anterior descending artery. Chest leads V1–V5 reflect electrical activity in the anterior myocardial wall, which is supplied by the left anterior descending artery. Usually, the inferior myocardial wall is supplied by the right coronary artery and the circumflex supplies the posterolateral wall.

   Essential Revision Notes for MRCP, 2nd edn, p 38

2. **E: Left lateral rectus**

   The effects of oculomotor mononeuropathies can be predicted using three rules: first, paresis of horizontally acting muscles causes predominantly horizontal diplopia, and of vertical muscles causes predominantly vertical diplopia. Second, the direction in which the separation of the two images is maximal is the direction of action of the weak muscle. Third, covering the affected eye leads to disappearance of the outer (false) image. In this case, these together suggest a left lateral rectus palsy.

   Essential Revision Notes for MRCP, 2nd edn, p 560

3. B: Right occipital lobe

Homonymous field defects (ie the same pattern in each eye) result from retrochiasmal lesions. Each visual field is represented contralaterally in the lateral geniculate nucleus, optic radiations and visual cortex. The superior optic radiation, which cuts through the deep white matter of the parietal lobe, carries the contralateral *inferior* visual field, whereas the inferior optic radiation carries the superior visual field. Consequently, parietal and temporal lesions can be associated with contralateral quadrantanopias. Here, the most likely cause of a left homonymous hemianopia is damage to the right occipital lobe.

Essential Revision Notes for MRCP, 2nd edn, p 556

4. E: Ulnar nerve

The ulnar nerve is derived from the C8 and T1 roots; in the hand it innervates the hypothenar muscles, the third and fourth lumbricals, the interossei and the adductor pollicis. Sensory supply is to the fifth finger, the ulnar aspect of the fourth finger and the ulnar border of the palm. The ulnar nerve may be damaged by pressure in the axilla, eg from the use of crutches, but is more commonly damaged at the elbow by trauma. Complete ulnar palsy results in a characteristic claw-hand deformity with hyperextension of the fingers at the metacarpophalangeal joints and flexion at the interphalangeal joints, which is most pronounced on the ulnar aspect of the hand.

Essential Revision Notes for MRCP, 2nd edn, p 580

5. D: L2–3

The spinal cord typically ends at the lower border of L2–3, well above the most frequent lumbar level for a lumbar puncture (L4–5).

Essential Revision Notes for MRCP, 2nd edn, p 570

6. **B: Common peroneal**

The common peroneal nerve is motor to the peroneal and anterior tibial muscles, and damage therefore results in paralysis of dorsiflexion (leading to foot drop) and inability to evert the foot. A lesion above the lateral cutaneous branch results in anaesthesia over the anterolateral lower leg and dorsum of the foot.

Essential Revision Notes for MRCP, 2nd edn, p 580

7. **E: Optic nerve**

Monocular field defects are typically caused by pathology affecting the eye or optic nerve. At the optic chiasma, the classic field defect is a bitemporal hemianopia. Posterior to the optic chiasma, the optic tracts lead to the lateral geniculate nucleus and then to the calcarine sulcus (primary visual cortex) in the occipital lobe, via the optic radiations. Retrochiasmal lesions produce congruous (homonymous) field defects in each eye.

Essential Revision Notes for MRCP, 2nd edn, p 556

8. **E: Anterior spinal artery occlusion**

Sensation is carried in the spinal cord posteriorly in the dorsal columns (vibration and joint position sense) and laterally in the spinothalamic tracts (pain and temperature). The anterior spinal artery supplies the ventral (anterior) two-thirds of the spinal cord, and so occlusion leads to leg weakness caused by ischaemia of the corticospinal tracts, loss of pain and temperature sensation below the lesion, but relatively preserved dorsal column sensation. It is associated with atherosclerosis and aortic aneurysm.

Essential Revision Notes for MRCP, 2nd edn, p 570

9. A: Middle cerebral artery

The middle and anterior cerebral arteries are formed from the terminal bifurcation of the internal carotid artery. The anterior cerebral arteries supply the medial surface of the frontal and parietal lobes, whereas the middle cerebral arteries supply the lateral surface of the cerebral hemispheres. A middle cerebral artery infarction will therefore typically cause hemiplegia, whereas an anterior cerebral artery infarction may cause leg weakness out of proportion to arm weakness as a result of the organisation of the motor homunculus. The posterior cerebral arteries derive from the basilar artery (which is, in turn, formed from the vertebral arteries) and supply the occipital lobe. The posterior inferior cerebellar artery is a branch of the vertebral artery.

Essential Revision Notes for MRCP, 2nd edn, p 572

10. C: Idiopathic pulmonary fibrosis

All of these disorders can be associated with reticulonodular shadowing on the chest X-ray, but typically affect the upper zone, with the exception of idiopathic pulmonary fibrosis.

Essential Revision Notes for MRCP, 2nd edn, p 683

11. B: Dorsum of foot

This is the clinical picture of a common peroneal nerve lesion (see Question 6) and so sensory loss in the distribution of this nerve, over the dorsum of the foot between the big and second toes, would be expected.

Essential Revision Notes for MRCP, 2nd edn, p 580

12. D: Intention tremor

Unilateral cerebellar hemisphere lesions can give rise to ipsilateral limb ataxia and intention tremor, together with (in varying combinations) hypotonia, dysdiadochokinesis, dysarthria and nystagmus. Astereognosis results most commonly from parietal lesions, damage to primary motor cortex can cause hemiparesis, and athetosis is a sinuous writhing movement associated with basal ganglia pathology, as is the rigidity often associated with Parkinson's disease.

Essential Revision Notes for MRCP, 2nd edn, p 551

13. E: δ Cells

The pancreas contains several different cell types. Islets of Langerhans are heavily vascularised groups of cells that constitute the endocrine pancreas. The most common cell type in the islets are the β cells, which produce insulin. α Cells produce glucagon and δ cells somatostatin.

Essential Revision Notes for MRCP, 2nd edn, p 178

14. C: Right upper zone

About 0.5% of routine chest X-rays will reveal an azygos lobe, which is a normal variant of the upper right lung developing around the azygos vein. On a chest X-ray the 'reverse comma sign' is seen, which extends in a curvilinear fashion towards the top of the right lung. The azygos lobe is not a true lobe with a separate segmental bronchus.

15. D: Median nerve

The median nerve is sensory to the lateral three and a half digits, mainly on the palmar side, whereas the ulnar nerve is sensory to the medial one and a half digits. The radial nerve is sensory to parts of the dorsal surface of the hand.

Essential Revision Notes for MRCP, 2nd edn, p 580

16. D: Rectum

Both ulcerative colitis and Crohn's disease are chronic relapsing inflammatory diseases of the gastrointestinal tract. Although Crohn's disease can affect any part of the gastrointestinal tract (most commonly the terminal ileum, colon or anorectum), ulcerative colitis always involves the rectum and extends back into the colon.

Essential Revision Notes for MRCP, 2nd edn, p 201

17. B: Weakness of the forehead muscles

The facial nerve is motor to the muscles of facial expression and stapedius, secretomotor to the parotid, submandibular and sublingual glands, and carries taste from the palate and anterior two-thirds of the tongue. A lesion at the geniculate ganglion will cause hyperacusis as a result of interruption of motor outflow to stapedius, loss of taste (not sensation) on the tongue, weakness of all the facial muscles (forehead muscles are spared in an upper motor neuron lesion of the nerve), but no change in lacrimation because the secretomotor portion of the facial nerve has already branched off.

Essential Revision Notes for MRCP, 2nd edn, p 566

18. C: Inability to adduct the thumb

The ulnar nerve in the forearm is motor to flexor carpi ulnaris and the ulnar (medial) half of flexor digitorum profundus. In the hand it is motor to the adductor pollicis muscle, all the muscles of the hypothenar eminence, the medial two lumbricals and all the interosseous muscles. Finger extension requires an intact radial nerve, which is also sensory to the dorsal aspect of the fingers (except the very tip). In the hand, the median nerve is motor to the lateral two lumbricals and all the muscles of the thenar eminence except adductor pollicis.

Essential Revision Notes for MRCP, 2nd edn, p 580

19. C: Lewy bodies

Lewy bodies are cytoplasmic inclusions that are classically described in neurons in the substantia nigra in patients with idiopathic Parkinson's disease. Lewy bodies found in cortical cells are associated with Lewy body dementia. The relationship between Lewy body dementia and Parkinson's disease is controversial. The former is characterised by progressive decline in cognitive function, but is specifically associated with substantial fluctuations in cognitive function, visual hallucinations and parkinsonian motor features. Patients are often exquisitely sensitive to small doses of neuroleptics for unknown reasons.

Essential Revision Notes for MRCP, 2nd edn, p 544

20. E: Patent foramen ovale

A patent foramen ovale is an interatrial communication that normally closes shortly after birth. Paradoxical embolism is possible, where a venous thrombus migrates and enters the systemic circulation through a patent foramen ovale. This can lead to cerebrovascular ischaemic events, as here. The other cardiac abnormalities are not associated with paradoxical embolism.

Essential Revision Notes for MRCP, 2nd edn, p 24

21. A: Allergic bronchopulmonary aspergillosis

Causes of upper lobe fibrosis include silicosis, sarcoidosis, allergic bronchopulmonary aspergillosis, tuberculosis (TB) or ankylosing spondylitis. Lower lobe fibrosis can be caused by rheumatoid arthritis, scleroderma, paraquat poisoning or pneumoconiosis.

Essential Revision Notes for MRCP, 2nd edn, p 669

22. D: Common peroneal nerve

The combination of foot drop with sensory loss over the dorsum of the foot is highly suggestive of common peroneal nerve palsy. The common peroneal nerve is motor to the peroneal muscles, which evert the foot, and tibialis anterior, which dorsiflexes the foot. It is sensory to a small area on the dorsum of the foot.

Essential Revision Notes for MRCP, 2nd edn, p 580

23. A: Atrophy of the mammillary bodies

Wernicke encephalopathy describes the combination of ophthalmoplegia, ataxia and an acute confusional state, and is the result of acute thiamine deficiency. If persistent memory deficit ensues, this is known as the Wernicke–Korsakoff syndrome. Anatomically, lesions are apparent in the hypothalamus, thalamus, periaqueductal grey matter, colliculi and floor of the fourth ventricle. The mammillary bodies are classically involved in all cases.

Essential Revision Notes for MRCP, 2nd edn, p 633

24. D: Ulnar nerve

The ulnar nerve supplies the adductor pollicis, whereas the median nerve is motor to all the other muscles of the thenar eminence. *See* Question 4.

Essential Revision Notes for MRCP, 2nd edn, p 580

25. A: Parietal lobe

Visual extinction is one component of the neglect syndrome, often following a right hemisphere stroke that affects the parietal lobe. Patients with visual extinction respond well to stimuli presented unilaterally to confrontation, but typically fail to respond to or 'extinguish' stimuli on one side of space when presented bilaterally. Classically, left visual extinction is associated with right parietal stroke.

Essential Revision Notes for MRCP, 2nd edn, p 541

26. B: Proximal convoluted tubule

Nephrotoxic drugs can act at different sites in the kidney to cause acute renal failure. Aminoglycoside drugs primarily act on the proximal convoluted tubule. In contrast, gold, interferon-alfa and penicillamine can alter glomerular function, cephalosporins cause interstitial nephritis, and non-steroidal anti-inflammatory drugs (NSAIDs) and angiotensin-converting enzyme (ACE) inhibitors cause vasoconstriction.

Essential Revision Notes for MRCP, 2nd edn, p 478

27. B: Testicle

The body contains immunologically privileged sites, where allografts do not elicit immune rejection. Such sites include the brain, testis, eye and uterus. Immune responses are supressed in such immunologically privileged sites, from which lymphocytes are excluded.

28. A: Left common carotid

The Horner syndrome is caused by interruption of sympathetic innervation of the eye. Signs seen in all patients are ptosis and miosis. Impaired sweating of the *face* ipsilateral to the lesion results from lesions affecting second-order neurons (those that exit the spinal cord at T1 to ascend in the cervical sympathetic chain and synapse in the superior cervical ganglion at the level of the bifurcation of the common carotid artery). Below this level, sweating abnormalities are usually absent.

Essential Revision Notes for MRCP, 2nd edn, p 558

29. B: Supraspinatus

Supraspinatus tendinitis presents with a painful aching shoulder. Pain is aggravated by abduction and external rotation against resistance. The tendon is located between the acromion and the head of the humerus, and is the most lateral tendon of the rotator cuff group between the infraspinatus and subscapularis tendons. The other tendons listed here are in very different locations.

30. C: Tricuspid regurgitation

Inspiration increases flow through the right side of the heart and so enhances the sound of tricuspid regurgitation. In contrast, the Valsalva manoeuvre will decrease preload and thus reduce many systolic murmurs, except for mitral valve prolapse, which will be made louder.

Essential Revision Notes for MRCP, 2nd edn, p 20

31. D: Medulla

Unilateral failure of the soft palate to rise when saying 'ah', accompanied by deviation of the uvula contralaterally, may indicate a unilateral vagal nerve palsy. Symptomatically this can present with dysarthria and hoarseness. The nerve nucleus is located in the medulla.

Essential Revision Notes for MRCP, 2nd edn, p 570

32. B: Tail of pancreas

The psoas muscle and the spleen are posterior to the kidney, whereas the suprarenal lies superior to it. The tail of the pancreas overlies the left kidney, extending to touch the splenic flexure.

33. E: Right coronary

The combination of a tall R wave in V1 with ST depression in leads V1–V3 is suggestive of a posterior myocardial infarction, 60% of cases being caused by the right coronary artery.

Essential Revision Notes for MRCP, 2nd edn, p 39

34. C: Lymphocyte depleted

Although clinical staging is a more important guide to prognosis in Hodgkin's disease than histology, prognosis worsens through histological types from lymphocyte predominant (best prognosis) to lymphocyte depleted (worst prognosis)

Essential Revision Notes for MRCP, 2nd edn, p 288

35. B: Turner syndrome

Aortic coarctation is a narrowing of the aorta most commonly found just distal to the origin of the left subclavian artery. Aortic coarctation can be associated with congenital abnormalities of the aortic valve, such as a bicuspid aortic valve. However it is more common in Turner syndrome where it can occur in up to 35% of individuals.

Essential Revision Notes for MRCP, 2nd edn, p 26

36. C: Ileum

Vitamin B_{12} (cobalamin) binds to intrinsic factor, a glycoprotein produced by stomach parietal cells, and is absorbed by specific receptors in the distal ileum. The intrinsic factor–cobalamin complex is then secreted into the circulation and taken up by the bone marrow, liver and other cells types. Deficiency of vitamin B_{12} is most commonly the result of malabsorption.

Essential Revision Notes for MRCP, 2nd edn, p 420

Chapter 3

CLINICAL BIOCHEMISTRY AND METABOLISM

Questions

---

1. Which one of the following is the most likely biochemical abnormality in a patient with primary adrenal insufficiency?

- ☐ A Hyperkalaemia
- ☐ B Hypernatraemia
- ☐ C Hypokalaemia
- ☐ D Hypocalcaemia
- ☐ E Hypoglycaemia

2. In which one of the following situations are transferrin levels most likely to be reduced?

- ☐ A Oral contraceptive therapy
- ☐ B Pregnancy
- ☐ C Haemochromatosis
- ☐ D Viral hepatitis
- ☐ E Iron-deficiency anaemia

Answers on pages 63–76

3. A 37-year-old man is found to have a high serum cholesterol on routine screening. Which one of the following features is most likely to be consistent with familial hypercholesterolaemia?

- ☐ A Tuberous xanthomas
- ☐ B Serum cholesterol > 10 mmol/l
- ☐ C Impaired glucose tolerance
- ☐ D Tendon xanthomas
- ☐ E Xanthelasma

4. Which one of the following can cause hypomagnesaemia?

- ☐ A Chronic diarrhoea
- ☐ B Hypothyroidism
- ☐ C Chronic respiratory failure
- ☐ D Diabetic ketoacidosis
- ☐ E Rhabdomyolysis

5. Which one of the following biochemical findings are most likely in a patient with primary hyperparathyroidism?

- ☐ A High calcium and high vitamin D
- ☐ B Low calcium and low phosphate
- ☐ C High calcium and low phosphate
- ☐ D Low calcium and high phosphate
- ☐ E Normal calcium and high phosphate

6. Which one of the following is most likely to result in de prolactin levels?

- ☐ A Metoclopramide
- ☐ B Pituitary adenoma
- ☐ C Bromocriptine
- ☐ D Polycystic ovarian syndrome
- ☐ E Pregnancy

7. What are the most likely biochemical findings in a patient wi Wilson's disease?

- ☐ A Low serum copper, high urinary copper
- ☐ B Normal serum copper, high urinary copper
- ☐ C High serum copper, high urinary copper
- ☐ D Low serum copper, normal urinary copper
- ☐ E Normal serum copper, low urinary copper

8. Which one of the following is most likely to be accompanied by abnormal haem biosynthesis?

- ☐ A Acute intermittent porphyria
- ☐ B Chronic myeloid leukaemia
- ☐ C Vitamin B_{12} deficiency
- ☐ D Carbon monoxide poisoning
- ☐ E Sickle-cell trait

Answers on pages 63–76

Which one of the following disorders is most likely to result from deficiency of vitamin B_1?

- A Pernicious anaemia
- B Kwashiorkor
- C Marasmus
- D Beri-beri
- E Pellagra

10. Elevation of which one of the following proteins is most likely to be associated with a decreased risk of atherosclerosis?

- A HDL (high-density lipoprotein)
- B LDL (low-density lipoprotein)
- C VLDL (very-low-density lipoprotein)
- D Chylomicrons
- E Albumin

11. Which one of the following laboratory findings is most likely to support a diagnosis of adrenal insufficiency?

- A Hypoglycaemia
- B Neutrophilia
- C Hypernatraemia
- D Anaemia
- E Hypokalaemia

12. Which one of the following biochemical abnormalities is most likely in a patient with primary hyperparathyroidism?

- ☐ A Decreased alkaline phosphatase
- ☐ B Increased parathyroid hormone
- ☐ C Increased serum phosphate
- ☐ D Normal urinary calcium
- ☐ E Decreased serum calcium

13. Which one of the following substances is most likely to inhibit vasopressin (ADH) release?

- ☐ A Aspirin
- ☐ B Barbiturates
- ☐ C Nicotine
- ☐ D Alcohol
- ☐ E Cocaine

14. Which one of the following symptoms are most likely in a patient with craniopharyngioma?

- ☐ A Polyuria and polydipsia
- ☐ B Blurred vision
- ☐ C Peripheral paraesthesiae
- ☐ D Amenorrhoea
- ☐ E Galactorrhoea

Answers on pages 63–76

15. Which one of the following is most likely falsely to depress a serum amylase measurement in a patient with suspected acute pancreatitis?

- ☐ A Hypocalcaemia
- ☐ B Hypertrigylceridaemia
- ☐ C Hyperphosphataemia
- ☐ D Hypercalcaemia
- ☐ E Hypercholesterolaemia

16. In which one of the following conditions is bilirubin most likely to be found in the urine?

- ☐ A Glucose-6-phosphate dehydrogenase (G6PD) deficiency
- ☐ B Gilbert syndrome
- ☐ C Sepsis
- ☐ D Hypothyroidism
- ☐ E Intrahepatic cholestasis

17. A 37-year-old woman has episodic leg weakness in association with crampy abdominal pain. Which biosynthetic pathway is most likely to be deficient?

- ☐ A Glucose
- ☐ B Corticosteroids
- ☐ C Acetylcholine
- ☐ D Thyroxine
- ☐ E Haem

18. A 24-year-old vegan presents with unsteady gait, and is found to have mild proximal weakness, absent joint position sense in the lower limbs and upgoing plantars. What nutritional deficiency is most likely to be responsible?

- ☐ A Iron
- ☐ B Vitamin B_1
- ☐ C Vitamin B_{12}
- ☐ D Iodine
- ☐ E Folic acid

19. Which one of the following is most likely to give rise to resistance to erythropoietin treatment of anaemia?

- ☐ A Iron deficiency
- ☐ B Angiotensin-converting enzyme (ACE) inhibitors
- ☐ C Hypoparathyroidism
- ☐ D Erythropoietin antibodies
- ☐ E Hypokalaemia

20. Which one of the following is most likely to be associated with elevated thyroid-binding globulin (TBG) levels?

- ☐ A Old age
- ☐ B Nephrotic syndrome
- ☐ C Hepatic failure
- ☐ D Malnutrition
- ☐ E Pregnancy

Answers on pages 63–76

21. Which one of the following is most likely to be an early feature of salicylate poisoning?

- ☐ A Hyperkalaemia
- ☐ B Respiratory alkalosis
- ☐ C Hyponatraemia
- ☐ D Lactic acidosis
- ☐ E Acidic urine

22. In which one of the following conditions is serum total iron-binding capacity most likely to be elevated?

- ☐ A β-Thalassaemia
- ☐ B Chronic renal failure
- ☐ C Acute intermittent porphyria
- ☐ D Sideroblastic anaemia
- ☐ E Pregnancy

23. Which one of the following serum measurements is most likely to occur in an acute phase response?

- ☐ A Increased iron
- ☐ B Decreased interleukin-1 (IL-1)
- ☐ C Increased tumour necrosis factor (TNF)
- ☐ D Increased zinc
- ☐ E Decreased endotoxin

24. Which one of the following factors is most likely to be associated with decreased HDL levels?

- ☐ A Low triglyceride levels
- ☐ B Cigarette smoking
- ☐ C Alcohol
- ☐ D Oestrogens
- ☐ E Familial hyperlipoporteinaemia

25. A 75-year-old man in acute renal failure as a result of outflow obstruction from prostatic hypertrophy is catheterised and passes large volumes of urine for several days. What is the most likely resulting biochemical abnormality?

- ☐ A Hypernatraemia
- ☐ B Hypomagnesaemia
- ☐ C Hypertrigylceridaemia
- ☐ D Hypocalcaemia
- ☐ E Hypercalcaemia

26. A patient receiving total parenteral nutrition (TPN) becomes drowsy with deranged serum electrolytes. What is the most likely cause?

- ☐ A Hypocalcaemia
- ☐ B Hypercalcaemia
- ☐ C Hypernatraemia
- ☐ D Hypophosphataemia
- ☐ E Hypomagnesaemia

Answers on pages 63–76

27. Which one of the following secondary hyperlipidaemias is most likely to be associated with elevated triglycerides?

- ☐ A Nephrotic syndrome
- ☐ B Hypothyroidism
- ☐ C Diabetes mellitus
- ☐ D Cholestasis
- ☐ E Cigarette smoking

28. Which one of the following causes of elevated alkaline phosphatase (ALP) is most likely to be associated with elevated serum calcium?

- ☐ A Hyperparathyroidism
- ☐ B Fracture
- ☐ C Puberty
- ☐ D Osteogenic sarcoma
- ☐ E Osteomalacia

29. Which one of the following causes of metabolic acidosis is most likely to be associated with a normal anion gap?

- ☐ A Hepatic failure
- ☐ B Renal failure
- ☐ C Ketoacidosis
- ☐ D Lactic acidosis
- ☐ E Hypoaldosteronism

30. Which one of the following findings is most consistent with a diagnosis of Cushing syndrome?

☐ A Normal urinary free cortisol

☐ B Low ACTH

☐ C Elevated ACTH

☐ D Low urinary free cortisol

☐ E High aldosterone level

31. Which one of the following is a disorder of purine metabolism?

☐ A Alkaptonuria

☐ B Gout

☐ C Maple syrup urine disease

☐ D Cystinuria

☐ E Oxalosis

32. Which one of the following is most likely to cause an abnormally low glycated haemoglobin (HbA1c) level?

☐ A Thalassaemia

☐ B Presence of haemoglobin HbS

☐ C Presence of HbF

☐ D Type 2 diabetes mellitus

☐ E Uraemia

Answers on pages 63–76

33. Which one of the following can cause an artificially elevated serum potassium level?

- ☐ A Delayed separation of red cells
- ☐ B Acute renal failure
- ☐ C Metabolic acidosis
- ☐ D Hyperlipidaemia
- ☐ E Hypomagnesaemia

34. Which one of the following enzymes is most likely to show decreased activity in beri-beri?

- ☐ A Pyruvate kinase
- ☐ B Phosphohexose isomerase
- ☐ C Enolase
- ☐ D G6PD
- ☐ E Pyruvate dehydrogenase

35. Which one of the following hormones is most likely to rise during acute illness?

- ☐ A TSH (thyroid-stimulating hormone)
- ☐ B GH (growth hormone)
- ☐ C LH (luteinising hormone)
- ☐ D FSH (follicle-stimulating hormone)
- ☐ E Testosterone

36. Which one of the following disorders characterised by hormone resistance is most likely to result from a second messenger defect?

- ☐ A Nephrogenic diabetes insipidus
- ☐ B Type 2 diabetes mellitus
- ☐ C Vitamin-D-dependent rickets
- ☐ D Testicular feminisation syndrome
- ☐ E Pseudohypoparathyroidism

37. Which one of the following laboratory findings is most consistent with acute renal failure?

- ☐ A Respiratory alkalosis
- ☐ B Metabolic acidosis
- ☐ C Metabolic alkalosis
- ☐ D Respiratory acidosis
- ☐ E Normal pH

38. A person with diabetes taking tolbutamide and bendrofluazide presents with hyponatraemia, hypokalaemia and decreased plasma osmolality. What is the most likely cause for the hyponatraemia?

- ☐ A Hyporeninaemic hypoaldosteronism
- ☐ B Tolbutamide therapy
- ☐ C Bendrofluazide therapy
- ☐ D True SIADH (syndrome of inappropriate secretion of ADH)
- ☐ E Pseudohyponatraemia

Answers on pages 63–76

39. Which one of the following causes of secondary hyperlipidaemia is more likely to be associated with increased triglycerides rather than increased cholesterol?

☐ A Renal transplantation

☐ B Hypothyroidism

☐ C Chronic renal failure

☐ D Nephrotic syndrome

☐ E Cholestasis

40. In congenital adrenal hyperplasia secondary to 21-hydroxylase deficiency, plasma levels of which one of the following substances are most likely to be elevated?

☐ A Aldosterone

☐ B ACTH

☐ C Sodium

☐ D Cortisol

☐ E Cholesterol

41. Which one of the following substances is most likely to mediate the transmission of Creutzfeldt–Jakob disease (CJD) from generation to generation?

☐ A Carbohydrate

☐ B Protein

☐ C Mitochondrial DNA

☐ D Nuclear DNA

☐ E RNA

42. A 63-year-old woman presents with lethargy, cold intolerance and fatigue, and is found to have low serum free T_4 (thyroxine) and normal TSH. What is the most appropriate next test?

- ☐ A Thyroid biopsy
- ☐ B T_3 (triiodothyronine)
- ☐ C Magnetic resonance imaging (MRI) of the pituitary
- ☐ D Thyroid autoantibodies
- ☐ E Prolactin

43. Which one of the following biochemical abnormalities is most likely in tumour lysis syndrome?

- ☐ A Hypercalcaemia
- ☐ B Metabolic alkalosis
- ☐ C Hypokalaemia
- ☐ D Hypophosphataemia
- ☐ E Lactic acidosis

44. A 23-year-old woman weighing 43 kg presents with lethargy. She has hyponatraemia with a high urinary osmolality and a low urinary sodium. What is the most likely explanation for her hyponatraemia?

- ☐ A Addison's disease
- ☐ B Bulimia
- ☐ C Diuretic abuse
- ☐ D SIADH
- ☐ E Acute renal failure

Answers on pages 63–76

45. Which one of the following is a metabolic effect of insulin?

- ☐ A Decreased glucose utilisation
- ☐ B Increased proteolysis
- ☐ C Increased ketogenesis
- ☐ D Increased gluconeogenesis
- ☐ E Decreased lipolysis

46. Which one of the following is most likely to result from hypoglycaemia?

- ☐ A Increased glucagon secretion
- ☐ B Decreased cortisol secretion
- ☐ C Increased testosterone secretion
- ☐ D Decreased insulin secretion
- ☐ E Decreased growth hormone secretion

47. An obese patient with increased abdominal striae has an elevated midnight cortisol level. Which one of the following would best confirm the diagnosis of Cushing disease?

- ☐ A Low-dose dexamethasone suppression test
- ☐ B Synacthen test
- ☐ C 24-hour urinary cortisol collection
- ☐ D High-dose dexamethasone suppression test
- ☐ E Basal ACTH levels

48. A menopausal woman is commenced on hormone replacement therapy. Which one of the following statements will best describe her position in 5 years' time?

- ☐ A Increased risk of osteoporotic fracture
- ☐ B Increased risk of pulmonary thromboembolism
- ☐ C Reduced risk of myocardial infarction
- ☐ D Increased risk of Alzheimer's disease
- ☐ E Increased risk of bowel cancer

CLINICAL BIOCHEMISTRY AND METABOLISM

Answers

1. **A: Hyperkalaemia**

   Primary adrenal insufficiency is Addison's disease, and patients are hyperkalaemic, hyponatraemic and hypotensive as a result of aldosterone deficiency. Hyperpigmentation can be striking, and abnormalities of gastrointestinal function (eg anorexia, nausea and vomiting) are often the presenting complaint. Plasma ACTH (adrenocorticotrophic hormone) levels are high as a result of the low cortisol removing the usual negative feedback effects on the hypothalamus and pituitary.

2. **C: Haemochromatosis**

   Iron is carried in the plasma in the ferric (Fe^{3+}) form, attached to transferrin. This specific binding protein is normally around one-third saturated with iron. Transferrin levels are raised in pregnancy and iron-deficiency anaemia, with the oral contraceptive pill and in viral hepatitis. Levels are normal or reduced in haemochromatosis.

3. **D: Tendon xanthomas**

   Xanthomas are localised collections of foam cells, which are histiocytes containing cytoplasmic lipid material together with cholesterol. They are caused by any disorder with elevated lipids or cholesterol. Tendon xanthomas are virtually pathognomonic of familial hypercholesterolaemia, because the only other causes of tendon xanthomas are very rare indeed.

4. A: Chronic diarrhoea

Causes of hypomagnesaemia include severe diarrhoea, chronic dialysis, diuretic therapy, acute pancreatitis, chronic alcoholism, malabsorption and fistulae.

Essential Revision Notes for MRCP, 2nd edn, p 414

5. C: High calcium and low phosphate

Primary hyperparathyroidism is most commonly caused by a single or multiple parathyroid adenomas. Biochemically it is characterised by increased parathyroid hormone (PTH) leading to raised serum and urinary calcium, with reduced serum phosphate and increased alkaline phosphatase.

Essential Revision Notes for MRCP, 2nd edn, p 409

6. C: Bromocriptine

Prolactin is secreted by the anterior pituitary and elevated levels can be associated with pituitary adenomas, secondary amenorrhoea, hypothyroidism, polycystic ovarian syndrome and pregnancy. Antiemetics and phenothiazine drugs can also cause hyperprolactinaemia. In contrast, dopamine agonists such as bromocriptine tend to suppress prolactin levels.

Essential Revision Notes for MRCP, 2nd edn, p 123

7. C: High serum copper, high urinary copper

Wilson's disease is an autosomal recessive disorder that results in defective intrahepatic formation of caeruloplasmin, the principal transport protein for copper, necessary for successful biliary excretion. Total body and tissue copper levels rise as a result of failure of biliary excretion, and urinary copper excretion increases.

Essential Revision Notes for MRCP, 2nd edn, p 395

8. A: Acute intermittent porphyria

The porphyrias are a rare group of abnormalities of enzymes involved in the biosynthesis of haem; they lead to overproduction of the intermediate compounds called porphyrins. Excess porphyrin production can be acute or non-acute and takes place in the liver or bone marrow.

Essential Revision Notes for MRCP, 2nd edn, p 397

9. D: Beri-beri

Vitamin B_1 is thiamine and deficiency is most likely to result from alcoholism and/or dietary deficiency. Beri-beri can be either 'dry' (a symmetrical sensorimotor neuropathy) or 'wet' (congestive cardiac failure), and thiamine deficiency can also be associated with the Wernicke–Korsakoff syndrome.

Essential Revision Notes for MRCP, 2nd edn, p 420

10. A: HDL

There is a strong relationship between total and LDL-cholesterol and coronary heart disease (CHD), whereas high levels of HDL are protective. A total cholesterol:HDL ratio > 4.5 is associated with increased risk of CHD. Elevated triglycerides are also associated with increased cardiovascular risk.

Essential Revision Notes, 2nd edn, p 400

11. A: Hypoglycaemia

Spontaneous hypoadrenalism is most likely (in the UK) to be the result of Addison's disease, with autoimmune destruction of the adrenal glands. Biochemical findings include hyponatraemia, hyperkalaemia and hypoglycaemia; haematological findings include lymphocytosis and a normocytic anaemia. Formal diagnosis depends on demonstrating failure of plasma cortisol to rise > 550 nmol/l at 30 or 60 minutes after an intramuscular or intravenous injection of ACTH (this the 'short Synacthen' test).

Essential Revision Notes for MRCP, 2nd edn, p 141

12. B: Increased Parathyroid hormone

Primary hyperparathyroidism is most likely to be caused by parathyroid adenoma (~85%) or hyperplasia (~10%). Biochemical changes include increased parathyroid hormone, serum and urinary calcium, decreased serum phosphate and increased alkaline phosphatase. Treatment is by parathyroidectomy.

Essential Revision Notes for MRCP, 2nd edn, p 409

13. D: Alcohol

Antidiuretic hormone (ADH) is synthesised in the hypothalamus and released from the posterior pituitary. It is released in response to rising plasma osmolality and acts to concentrate the urine by increasing water reabsorption in the distal nephron. Nicotine acts to release ADH whereas alcohol inhibits ADH secretion. Other factors stimulating ADH secretion include acute hypoglycaemia and glucocorticoid deficiency. Drugs that increase ADH levels include aspirin, barbiturates, oral hypoglycaemic agents and tricyclic antidepressants.

Essential Revision Notes for MRCP, 2nd edn, p 128

14. A: Polyuria and polydipsia

Craniopharyngiomas are benign tumours that arise from embryonic remnants of Rathke's pouch. Most arise in the hypothalamus, and they not uncommonly present in adulthood with cranial diabetes insipidus, resulting in polyuria and polydipsia. They can also cause bitemporal hemianopia as with any pituitary tumour.

Essential Revision Notes for MRCP, 2nd edn, p 128

15. B: Hypertrigylceridaemia

During hypertriglyceridaemia, the serum can contain inhibitors that falsely depress amylase results.

Essential Revision Notes, 2nd edn, p 190

16. E: Intrahepatic cholestasis

Only conjugated bilirubin appears in the urine. The other options are all causes of pre-hepatic jaundice, which results in unconjugated hyperbilirubinaemia. Thus, in these cases bilirubin does not appear in the urine ('acholuric jaundice').

Essential Revision Notes for MRCP, 2nd edn, p 210

17. E: Haem

This question tests the clinical presentation corresponding to the knowledge of porphyrin biosynthesis tested in Question 8. Acute intermittent porphyria classically presents with intermittent episodic abdominal pain, neuropsychiatric disorders and motor neuropathy. Acute episodes are often precipitated by infection, drugs (especially barbiturates and sulphonamides), or normal fluctuations in female sex hormones.

Essential Revision Notes for MRCP, 2nd edn, p 398

18. C: Vitamin B_{12}

Vitamin B_{12} (cobalamin) binds to intrinsic factor in the stomach and is then absorbed in the terminal ileum (*see* Clinical Anatomy, Question 36). In this case, deficiency is likely to be dietary because most vitamin B_{12} is obtained from foods of animal origin. Neurological symptoms and signs arise from damage to the peripheral nerves and spinal cord, and include paraesthesiae, sensory loss, particularly affecting the dorsal columns, and upper motor neuron signs, including upgoing plantars.

Essential Revision Notes for MRCP, 2nd edn, p 181

19. A: Iron deficiency

Endogneous erythropoietin is normally synthesised by renal peritubular cells. Resistance to exogenous erythropoietin therapy (eg in renal dialysis patients) is associated with iron deficiency, sepsis, chronic inflammation or hyperparathyroidism. Pure red cell aplasia is an uncommon progressive severe anaemia that is associated with antibodies directed towards erythropoietin, but as it is so uncommon the best of the five options is Answer A.

Essential Revision Notes for MRCP, 2nd edn, p 486

20. E: Pregnancy

Thyroid-binding globulin is the protein that transports thyroid hormones around the body. Oestrogen therapy, pregnancy, phenothiazine therapy, heroin abuse, acute intermittent porphyria and HIV infection can all elevate TBG levels. Nephrotic syndrome, hepatic failure and malnutrition are more likely to decrease TBG levels.

Essential Revision Notes for MRCP, 2nd edn, p 122

21. B: Respiratory alkalosis

Salicylate poisoning leads to accumulation of organic acids, causing metabolic acidosis, but initially it causes alkalosis from direct stimulation of the respiratory centre in the brain stem. Other early symptoms include sweating and tinnitus; hypokalaemia may be evident on blood testing.

Essential Revision Notes for MRCP, 2nd edn, p 91

22. E: Pregnancy

Total iron-binding capacity (TIBC) is commonly elevated in iron-deficiency anaemia, and also in the later stages of pregnancy. Lowered TIBC is associated with cirrhosis, haemolytic anaemias, pernicious anaemia, sickle-cell disease, inflammation, malnutrition and hypoproteinaemic states.

Essential Revision Notes for MRCP, 2nd edn, p 274

23. C: Increased TNF

In addition to fever, the acute phase response is associated with alterations in gene regulation and metabolism in the liver. Fever is mediated through local generation of the cytokines IL-1, TNF-α and IL-6 at the site of tissue injury, leading to induction of the prostaglandin PGE_2. In the liver, acute phase reactants are then generated including serum amyloid A, C-reactive protein (CRP) and many other proteins.

Essential Revision Notes for MRCP, 2nd edn, p 448

24. B: Cigarette smoking

Increased HDL levels are protective against cardiovascular disease. All of the options act to increase HDL levels with the exception of cigarette smoking. HDL levels are also decreased with hypertriglyceridaemia, obesity and diabetes mellitus.

Essential Revision Notes for MRCP, 2nd edn, p 402

25. B: Hypomagnesaemia

When bladder obstruction is relieved, polyuria is likely to result with excretion of a hypotonic urine containing large amounts of sodium, potassium and magnesium. Excretion of retained urea also promotes an osmotic diuresis. Hyponatraemia and hypomagnesaemia are most common, but excessive loss of water can also less commonly lead to hypernatraemia, essentially as a result of a nephrogenic diabetes insipidus.

26. C: Hypernatraemia

Metabolic complications of TPN can include many different electrolyte abnormalities, related either to the underlying disorder requiring TPN or to the TPN therapy itself. Hypocalcaemia is likely to lead to: muscle cramps, confusion and seizures rather than drowsiness; hypercalcaemia leads to anorexia, nausea and vomiting, hypomagnesaemia to neuromuscular hyperactivity and cardiac arrhythmia, and hypophosphataemia to irritability. Hypernatraemia can cause restlessness and irritability followed by drowsiness and coma.

27. C: Diabetes mellitus

Secondary triglyceridaemias are usually mixed (cholesterol and triglycerides both elevated), but elevated triglycerides predominate in alcoholism, chronic renal failure and diabetes mellitus, whereas cholesterol is predominantly increased in nephritic syndrome, hypothyroidism and cholestasis, and in association with cigarette smoking.

Essential Revision Notes for MRCP, 2nd edn, p 403

28. A: Hyperparathyroidism

Elevated ALP can occur with low, normal or high calcium. Hyperparathyroidism is specially associated with elevated calcium and elevated ALP. Fracture is associated with a normal calcium; elevated ALP is associated with puberty and osteogenic sarcoma. Serum calcium is usually low in osteomalacia.

Essential Revision Notes for MRCP, 2nd edn, p 412

29. E: Hypoaldosteronism

The anion gap represents the level of unmeasured anions in the plasma and is calculated as the plasma sodium concentration minus the sum of the chloride and bicarbonate concentrations. An increased anion gap associated with metabolic acidosis indicates the presence of unmeasured anions such as acetoacetate or lactate, or uraemic organic anions. Thus lactic acidosis, diabetic ketoacidosis, lactic acidosis and acute or chronic renal failure are associated with a high anion-gap acidosis (also salicylate poisoning). Hypoaldosteronism causes a metabolic acidosis with a normal anion gap.

Essential Revision Notes for MRCP, 2nd edn, p 421

30. B: Low ACTH

Cushing syndrome is due to prolonged excess elevated levels of circulating glucocorticoids, resulting from either exogenously administered glucocorticoids or by endogenous over-production of cortisol. There are elevated levels of urinary free cortisol. ACTH can either be low (suggestive of a primary adrenal tumour, or consistent with exogenous administration of steroids with suppression of the pituitary-adrenal axis) or elevated (suggestive of an ACTH dependent pituitary adenoma). However, ACTH can also be elevated during acute illness; and as exogenous administration of steroids is the commonest cause of Cushing syndrome, a low ACTH is most consistent in this case.

Essential Revision Notes for MRCP, 2nd edn, pp 138–9

31. B: Gout

Hyperuricaemia can have a number of causes, but when it leads to uric acid crystals forming in joints or soft tissues then gout can result. Uric acid arises as a breakdown of purine nucleotides, which are both a part of the normal diet and released at cell death. Gout can therefore result from either a primary or secondary hyperuricaemia; examples of the latter include myeloproliferative disorders, dietary excess or renal failure.

Essential Revision Notes for MRCP, 2nd edn, p 393

32. B: Presence of HbS

Abnormally low HbA1c can arise from any cause of increased red cell turnover or haemolysis, blood loss or the presence of HbS or HbC. In contrast, abnormally high HbA1c levels can be asssociated with persistent HbF (fetal haemoglobin), thalassaemia or during uraemia.

Essential Revision Notes for MRCP, 2nd edn, p 154

33. A: Delayed separation of red cells

Artefactually high potassium levels can be caused by haemolysis (eg from filling a Vacutainer from a syringe, exposing a specimen to heat and light), passive leakage of potassium (through leaving the sample for several hours before analysis) or contamination. Pseudohyperkalaemia is caused by passive leakage of potassium from cells. Causes include haemolysis (some inherited conditions), marked leucocytosis or thrombocytosis (eg myeloproliferative disorders), or prolonged use of a tourniquet.

34. E: Pyruvate dehydrogenase

Beri-beri results from thiamine (vitamin B_1) deficiency. Thiamine in its active form works as a coenzyme in a number of important reactions in the citrate cycle, including the conversion of pyruvate to acetyl-CoA, which is catalysed by pyruvate dehydrogenase within mitochondria.

35. B: GH

In acute illness or stress the hypothalamic–pituitary–adrenocortical axis is activated, with enhanced secretion of GH and prolactin, the presence of low circulating levels of insulin-like growth factor I (IGF-I), suppressed thyroid activity and a suppressed gonadal axis. These endocrine changes reduce energy consumption and anabolism, and activate the immune response.

36. E: Pseudohypoparathyroidism

Hormone resistance syndromes are characterised by impaired response of end-organs to a hormone, and have a number of underlying mechanisms including second messenger deficits. Pseudohypoparathyroidism was the first described example of a hormone resistance syndrome caused by renal unresponsiveness to parathyroid hormone, proximal to generation of the second messenger cAMP.

Essential Revision Notes for MRCP, 2nd edn, p 120

37. C: Metabolic alkalosis

Acute renal failure is associated with a decreased plasma pH and a high anion-gap metabolic acidosis (*see* Question 29) caused by accumulation of endogenous acids.

Essential Revision Notes for MRCP, 2nd edn, p 474

38. B: Tolbutamide therapy

Serum osmolality is normal in pseudohyponatraemia (ie from hyperlipidaemia or hyperproteinaemia). SIADH has many causes, but thiazide diuretics cause renal sodium loss (by impairing diluting capacity without limiting concentrating ability) and tolbutamide potentiates the action of ADH. The combination of therapies is therefore the most likely cause of the SIADH described here.

Essential Revision Notes for MRCP, 2nd edn, p 132

39. C: Chronic renal failure

End-stage renal failure is commonly associated with mild hypertriglyceridaemia caused by accumulation of VLDLs in the circulation. Similarly, patients who are recipients of renal transplants are usually hyperlipidaemic as a result of immunosuppressive drugs such as glucocorticoids and ciclosporin. In contrast, nephrotic syndrome is usually associated with a mixed hyperlipidaemia, and hypothyroidism and cholestasis with hypercholesterolaemia.

Essential Revision Notes for MRCP, 2nd edn, p 402

40. B: ACTH

Deficiency of 21-hydoxylase causes a block in adrenal glucocorticoid (eg cortisol) and mineralocorticoid (eg aldosterone) synthesis, shunting precursors into the androgen synthesis pathway. This leads to compensatory elevation of ACTH as a result of the lowered levels of glucocorticoids.

Essential Revision Notes for MRCP, 2nd edn, p 140–1

41. D: Nuclear DNA

Intergenerational transfer of this prion disease occurs via point mutations in the gene coding for prion protein on chromosome 22. This transmembrane protein is conformationally changed in disease, and can act as an infectious agent for transmission between people (eg dural grafts, cadaver-associated pituitary hormones) or between species (eg bovine spongiform encephalopathy [BSE] and new variant CJD [nvCJD]).

Essential Revision Notes for MRCP, 2nd edn, p 451

42. C: MRI of the pituitary

The serum TSH level is the key to distinguishing primary and secondary hypothyroidism. A low free T_4 in association with an elevated TSH suggests primary hypothyroidism, whereas pituitary or hypothalamic disease is suggested by a low free T_4 in the absence of TSH elevation (although note that critical illness, and some medications, eg dopamine, can impair the normal response of TSH to hypothyroxinaemia). An MRI of the pituitary is therefore the best investigation.

43. E: Lactic acidosis

Tumour lysis syndrome can occur during chemotherapy when large numbers of tumour cells are rapidly killed, leading to the release of large amounts of intracellular potassium, phosphate and nucleic acids. This in turn leads to hyperphosphataemia, hyperkalaemia and lactic acidosis. There is hypocalcaemia as a result of the hyperphosphataemia, which may result in tetany. Acute renal failure may also result.

44. B: Bulimia

A high urine osmolality indicates that water excretion is impaired. ADH excess, cortisol deficiency (eg Addison's disease), acute renal failure and abuse of diuretics would both cause excess urinary sodium loss. Coupled with her low weight, the most likely diagnosis here is bulimia.

45. E: Decreased lipolysis

Insulin affects the metabolism of carbohydrates, proteins and lipids. It causes hypoglycaemia by increasing tissue uptake of glucose and by inhibiting hepatic glucose release. It promotes glycogen formation and inhibits gluconeogenesis. Insulin decreases proteolysis and increases tissue uptake of amino acids. Insulin promotes lipogenesis and inhibits lipolysis.

46. A: Increased glucagon secretion

Glucagon is secreted when blood glucose falls. This stimulates hepatic release of glucose, and also promotes gluconeogenesis. Cortisol and growth hormone production is stimulated.

47. D: High-dose dexamethasone suppression test

Cushing's disease is caused by an ACTH-secreting pituitary adenoma and results in Cushing's sydrome. Cushing's syndrome can be diagnosed by demonstrating increased cortisol production (eg 24h urinary free cortisol) and failure to suppress cortisol secretion normally when low-dose dexamethasone is administered. High dose dexamethasone suppression tests are useful in distinguishing Cushing's disease (a ACTH-secreting) pituitary adenoma from other forms of Cushing's syndrome, as here.

48. B: Increased risk of pulmonary thromboembolism

Hormone replacement therapy will not only improve menopausal symptoms but also protect against fracture secondary to osteoporosis. There may be reduced incidence of Alzheimer's disease and colon cancer, but there may be increased risk of deep venous thrombosis and pulmonary embolism.

Chapter 4
CLINICAL PHYSIOLOGY
Questions

---

1. Which one of the following increases the affinity of haemoglobin for oxygen?

☐ A Carbon monoxide poisoning

☐ B Increased levels of 2,3-diphosphoglycerate (DPG)

☐ C Exercise

☐ D Metabolic acidosis

☐ E High temperature

2. Spirometry in a 57-year-old man shows a reduction in FEV_1 (forced expiratory volume in 1 s) with a preserved FVC (forced vital capacity). Which one of the following diagnoses is most likely?

☐ A Pleural effusion

☐ B Obesity

☐ C Myasthenia gravis

☐ D Pulmonary fibrosis

☐ E Asthma

Answers on pages 95–108

3. Which one of the following is most likely to be consistent with a diagnosis of established tubular necrosis?

- ☐ A Urine:plasma urea ratio of 10:1
- ☐ B Proteinuria 3.2 g/day
- ☐ C Urinary osmolality < 320 mosmol/kg
- ☐ D Elevated C-reactive protein (CRP)
- ☐ E Urinary sodium < 20 mmol/l

4. Which one of the following is a feature of methaemoglobinaemia?

- ☐ A Normal oxygen saturation levels
- ☐ B Metabolic acidosis
- ☐ C Cyanosis responding to oxygen administration
- ☐ D Respiratory alkalosis
- ☐ E Hypocalcaemia

5. Which one of the following spinal pathways is most likely to carry signals related to pain?

- ☐ A Spinocerebellar tract
- ☐ B Pyramidal tract
- ☐ C Spinothalamic tract
- ☐ D Dorsal columns
- ☐ E Medial lemniscus

6. In the evaluation of a patient with renal failure, which one of the following test results makes pre-renal failure relatively unlikely?

- ☐ A Urinary osmolality > 500 mosmol/l
- ☐ B Urinary sodium > 20 mmol/l
- ☐ C Urine:plasma urea ratio > 8
- ☐ D Postural hypotension
- ☐ E Hyponatraemia

7. Which one of the following is most likely to be associated with a prolonged bleeding time?

- ☐ A Thrombocytopenia
- ☐ B Protein C deficiency
- ☐ C Protein S deficiency
- ☐ D Factor IX deficiency
- ☐ E Factor VIII deficiency

8. What is the primary neurotransmitter deficiency in idiopathic Parkinson's disease?

- ☐ A Substance P
- ☐ B γ-Aminobutyric acid
- ☐ C Dopamine
- ☐ D Acetylcholine
- ☐ E Glutamate

Answers on pages 95–108

9. Which one of the following substances is activated by passage within the lung?

- ☐ A Angiotensin I
- ☐ B Serotonin
- ☐ C Epinephrine (adrenaline)
- ☐ D Bradykinin
- ☐ E Histamine

10. In a patient admitted to hospital with diabetic ketoacidosis, which one of the following is most likely to be elevated?

- ☐ A Arterial $P\text{CO}_2$
- ☐ B Plasma pH
- ☐ C Serum bicarbonate concentration
- ☐ D Anion gap
- ☐ E Arterial $P\text{O}_2$

11. Which one of the following is most likely to cause hyperprolactinaemia?

- ☐ A Corticosteroids
- ☐ B Haloperidol
- ☐ C Thyroxine
- ☐ D Phenytoin
- ☐ E Bromocriptine

12. Which one of the following factors is most likely to increase cerebral blood flow?

- ☐ A Polycythaemia
- ☐ B Hypothermia
- ☐ C Decreased arterial $P\text{CO}_2$
- ☐ D Tachypnoea
- ☐ E Grand mal seizure

13. Which one of the following findings on electromyography (EMG) would be most suggestive of active denervation?

- ☐ A Slow motor conduction velocity
- ☐ B Short duration motor unit potentials
- ☐ C Positive sharp waves
- ☐ D Motor conduction block
- ☐ E Increased F-wave latency

14. Which one of the following types of peripheral nerve will have the greatest conduction velocity?

- ☐ A Large unmyelinated nerve
- ☐ B Small unmyelinated nerve
- ☐ C Large myelinated nerve
- ☐ D Small myelinated nerve
- ☐ E None; all have the same velocity

Answers on pages 95–108

15. A woman presents with dyspnoea and left tracheal deviation secondary to a retrosternal goitre. What is the best respiratory function test parameter to demonstrate her upper airway obstruction?

☐ A Flow–volume loop

☐ B FEV_1

☐ C FVC

☐ D PEFR (peak expiratory flow rate)

☐ E RV (residual volume)

16. Which one of the following conditions is most likely to be associated with J waves on the ECG?

☐ A Hypocalcaemia

☐ B Hypothermia

☐ C Hypokalaemia

☐ D Hyponatraemia

☐ E Hypothyroidism

17. Which one of the following measurements will be greater at the lung apex when standing?

☐ A Ventilation

☐ B Perfusion

☐ C Lung compliance

☐ D Ventilation–perfusion ratio

☐ E $P\text{CO}_2$

18. During adaptation to altitude, which one of the following will return to normal?

- ☐ A Arterial oxygen tension
- ☐ B Arterial bicarbonate concentration
- ☐ C Arterial pH
- ☐ D Erythropoietin levels
- ☐ E Haemoglobin concentration

19. Which one of the following tests is most likely to be used to determine the cause of vitamin B_{12} deficiency?

- ☐ A Lactose tolerance test
- ☐ B Schilling's test
- ☐ C Schirmer's test
- ☐ D Glucose tolerance test
- ☐ E Wada test

20. Which one of the following physical signs is most consistent with a diagnosis of cardiac tamponade?

- ☐ A Systolic murmur
- ☐ B Third heart sound
- ☐ C Hypertension
- ☐ D Pulsus paradoxus
- ☐ E Bradycardia

21. Which one of the following substances is most likely to cause peripheral vasodilation?

- ☐ A Prostaglandin
- ☐ B Anaemia
- ☐ C ADP
- ☐ D Nitric oxide
- ☐ E Endothelin

22. Which one of the following is most likely to stimulate renin release?

- ☐ A Anaemia
- ☐ B Hypertension
- ☐ C Hyperkalaemia
- ☐ D Hypotension
- ☐ E Hypernatraemia

23. Cyanosis is most likely to be a feature of which one of the following disorders?

- ☐ A Eisenmenger syndrome
- ☐ B Aortic stenosis
- ☐ C Patent ductus arteriosus (PDA)
- ☐ D Pulmonary stenosis
- ☐ E Ostium primum atrial septal defect (ASD)

24. Which one of the following hormones is most likely to stimulate the emptying of the stomach?

- ☐ A Cholecystokinin
- ☐ B Leptin
- ☐ C Somatostatin
- ☐ D Glucagon
- ☐ E Gastrin

25. Which one of the following is most likely as a sustained response during the Valsalva manoeuvre?

- ☐ A Decreased intrathoracic pressure
- ☐ B Bradycardia
- ☐ C Elevated blood pressure
- ☐ D Tachycardia
- ☐ E Decreased JVP

26. What is the QRS complex on the ECG most likely to correspond to?

- ☐ A Interventricular conduction
- ☐ B Ventricular repolarisation
- ☐ C Atrial contraction
- ☐ D Isovolumetric contraction
- ☐ E Ventricular emptying

27. Which one of the following ECG changes is most likely to be seen in hyperkalaemia?

- ☐ A Prolonged P–R interval
- ☐ B Shortened P–R interval
- ☐ C ST depression
- ☐ D Flat T waves
- ☐ E Inverted T waves

28. Which one of the following is most likely to represent a normal physiological change in pregnancy?

- ☐ A Decreased thyroxine (T_4)
- ☐ B Decreased triiodothyronine (T_3)
- ☐ C Increased thyroxine-binding globulin (TBG)
- ☐ D Elevated T_4:T_3 ratio
- ☐ E Elevated thyroid-stimulating hormone (TSH)

29. Which one of the following factors is most likely to inhibit renin release?

- ☐ A Interleukins
- ☐ B Prostaglandins
- ☐ C β-Adrenergic agonists
- ☐ D Decreased sympathetic activity
- ☐ E Aldosterone

30. Which one of the following is most likely to lead to increased release of calcium from bone?

- ☐ A Increased osteocyte activity
- ☐ B Hyperphosphataemia
- ☐ C Hypercalcaemia
- ☐ D Decreased osteoblast activity
- ☐ E Increased osteoclast activity

31. Which one of the following changes is most likely to result from congestive cardiac failure?

- ☐ A Increased tumour necrosis factor α (TNF-α)
- ☐ B Increased calcitonin gene-related peptide (CGRP)
- ☐ C Decreased endothelin
- ☐ D Decreased atrial natriuretic peptide (ANP)
- ☐ E Decreased antidiuretic hormone (ADH)

32. Which one of the following hormones inhibits gastric acid secretion?

- ☐ A Vasoactive intestinal peptide (VIP)
- ☐ B Cholecystokinin
- ☐ C Gastrin
- ☐ D Leptin
- ☐ E Somatostatin

Answers on pages 95–108

33. Which one of the following is most likely to be a feature of carbon monoxide poisoning?

- ☐ A Increased arterial $P\text{O}_2$
- ☐ B Decreased arterial $P\text{O}_2$
- ☐ C Decreased arterial $P\text{CO}_2$
- ☐ D Increased affinity of haemoglobin for oxygen
- ☐ E Decreased affinity of haemoglobin for oxygen

34. Which one of the following physiological changes is most likely to be seen in pulmonary emphysema?

- ☐ A Increased vital capacity
- ☐ B Increased pulmonary compliance
- ☐ C Increased elastic recoil pressure
- ☐ D Increased diffusivity coefficient for carbon monoxide
- ☐ E Normal FEV_1

35. Which one of the following factors is most likely to lead to increased renin release?

- ☐ A ANP
- ☐ B Angiotensin II
- ☐ C Hypernatraemia
- ☐ D Vasopressin
- ☐ E Hyponatraemia

36. Which one of the following investigations is the most appropriate screening investigation for diabetic nephropathy?

- ☐ A Creatinine clearance
- ☐ B Serum creatinine level
- ☐ C Urinary albumin
- ☐ D Oral glucose tolerance test
- ☐ E Renal ultrasonography

37. Which one of the following effects will result from increased production of ANP?

- ☐ A Decreased renal excretion of sodium
- ☐ B Increased aldosterone
- ☐ C Increased renin release
- ☐ D Increased renal blood flow
- ☐ E Reduced stroke volume

38. Which one of the following physiological changes is most likely in pregnancy?

- ☐ A Decreased blood volume
- ☐ B Decreased hepatic blood flow
- ☐ C Increased renal blood flow
- ☐ D Increased total peripheral resistance
- ☐ E Decreased cardiac output

39. Which one of the following conditions is most likely to result in hyperphosphataemia secondary to increased tubular reabsorption of phosphate?

- ☐ A Renal failure
- ☐ B Tumour lysis syndrome
- ☐ C Rhabdomyolysis
- ☐ D Lactic acidosis
- ☐ E Hypoparathyroidism

40. What is the most likely effect of increased parasympathetic nervous system activity on the cardiovascular system?

- ☐ A Decreased heart rate
- ☐ B Increased contractility
- ☐ C Increased conduction velocity
- ☐ D Decreased arteriolar resistance
- ☐ E Increased stroke volume

41. In a patient with COPD suffering an acute infective exacerbation, which one of the following features would be most likely to suggest suitability for non-invasive forms of ventilatory support?

- ☐ A Acute confusional state
- ☐ B Decreased level of consciousness
- ☐ C Severe hypoxia
- ☐ D Severe hypercapnia without significant hypoxia
- ☐ E Carbon monoxide poisoning

42. Which one of the following laboratory findings is most likely to be seen after a pulmonary embolism?

- ☐ A Elevated serum troponin
- ☐ B Reduced serum lactate level
- ☐ C Reduced white cell count
- ☐ D Elevated arterial $P\text{CO}_2$
- ☐ E Normal serum D-dimer

43. A 48-year-old man presents with a broad complex tachycardia. Which one of the following features is most likely to confirm a diagnosis of ventricular tachycardia?

- ☐ A Discordant chest lead polarity
- ☐ B Absence of fusion beats
- ☐ C QRS duration of < 140 ms
- ☐ D Absence of capture beats
- ☐ E Independent P-wave activity

44. Lung function tests for a breathless 70-year-old reveal a decreased FEV_1, decreased FVC, relatively preserved FEV_1:FVC ratio and decreased transfer factor. Which one of the following diagnoses is most likely?

- ☐ A Pleural effusion
- ☐ B Kyphoscoliosis
- ☐ C Sarcoidosis
- ☐ D Bronchiectasis
- ☐ E COPD

Answers on pages 95–108

45. Which one of the following is most likely to remain in the normal range in a patient with obstructive liver disease?

☐ A ALP

☐ B Conjugated bilirubin

☐ C γGT (γ-glutamyl transferase)

☐ D Unconjugated bilirubin

☐ E Aspartate transaminase (AST)

46. Which one of the following is most likely to occur during normal inspiration?

☐ A Negative intrathoracic pressure

☐ B Positive intrathoracic pressure

☐ C Fall in diaphragm of 10 cm

☐ D Rise in diaphragm of 10 cm

☐ E Contraction of abdominal muscles

47. A 68-year-old presents with recurrent diarrhoea, weight loss and easy bruising. Blood tests reveal a prolonged prothrombin time. Which one of the following vitamins is most likely to be deficient?

☐ A Vitamin A

☐ B Vitamin B_{12}

☐ C Vitamin D

☐ D Vitamin E

☐ E Vitamin K

48. Which one of the following statements is correct about the physiological changes introduced by intubation and mechanical ventilation?

- ☐ A Lung volumes are decreased
- ☐ B Pulmonary vascular resistance is decreased
- ☐ C Cardiac output falls
- ☐ D Intrathoracic blood volume increases
- ☐ E Systemic blood pressure increases

CLINICAL PHYSIOLOGY

Answers

1. A: Carbon monoxide poisoning

The oxyhaemoglobin dissociation curve is sigmoid in shape and describes the affinity of haemoglobin for oxygen. The curve is shifted to the right (decreased affinity, increased tissue offloading) by high temperature, acidosis, increased $P\text{CO}_2$ and increased levels of 2,3-DPG. It is shifted to the left by opposite changes and the presence of carboxyhaemoglobin in carbon monoxide poisoning.

Essential Revision Notes for MRCP, 2nd edn, p 648

2. A: Pleural effusion

FEV_1 refers to the volume exhaled in the first second of a forced expiration, whereas FVC refers to the total volume exhaled on forced expiration. A reduction in FEV_1 with preserved FVC is characteristic of obstructive pulmonary disorders such as asthma or chronic obstructive pulmonary disease (COPD). In contrast, a reduction in FVC with preserved FEV_1:FVC ratio occurs in restrictive lung diseases such as pulmonary fibrosis.

Essential Revision Notes for MRCP, 2nd edn, p 645

3. C: Urinary osmolality < 320 mosmol/kg

Acute tubular necrosis results in failure of sodium reabsorption and tubular concentrating ability. Thus the urinary osmolality is low and urinary sodium relatively high. Pre-renal renal failure is more likely to lead to an elevated urine:plasma urea ratio and a low concentration of urinary sodium, whereas a high level of proteinuria is likely to suggest glomerular rather than tubular pathology.

4. A: Normal oxygen saturation levels

Methaemoglobinaemia is a condition where the iron within haemoglobin is oxidised from the ferrous to the ferric state, resulting in the inability to transport oxygen or carbon dioxide. The disorder can be congenital or acquired from exposure to oxidising substances (eg aniline dyes). Clinically, cyanosis occurs as a result of the presence of abnormal haemoglobin; as the cyanosis is not caused by deoxygenated haemoglobin, oxygen saturation can be normal and cyanosis does not respond to oxygen.

5. C: Spinothalamic tract

The two principal ascending pathways in the spinal cord that carry sensation are the dorsal (posterior) columns and the spinothalamic tracts. The dorsal columns carry signals related to joint position sense and vibration, and ascend ipsilateral to their origin until they synapse and then decussate in the brain stem. In contrast, the spinothalamic tracts carry signals related to pain and temperature sensation, and are crossed, ascending contralaterally.

6. B: Urine sodium > 20 mmol/l

Pre-renal failure results from poor renal perfusion, and the kidney retains sodium while excreting urea. Hence urinary sodium levels are low and urinary urea levels high, compared with the corresponding plasma levels. Urinary osmolality is high because a concentrated urine is excreted. Pre-renal failure is likely to be accompanied by other signs of volume depletion such as postural hypotension.

7. A: Thrombocytopenia

The bleeding time is a sensitive measure of platelet function, and is measured by timing the duration of bleeding from a standardised skin incision. Bleeding time can be prolonged as a result of either thrombocytopenia (usually with counts $< 100 \times 10^9$/l) or qualitative disorders of platelet function (eg von Willebrand's disease or after aspirin therapy).

8. C: Dopamine

Idiopathic Parkinson's disease is a disorder characterised by rigidity, bradykinesia and a resting tremor. It is a neurodegenerative disorder associated with loss of dopaminergic neurons in the substantia nigra (an area in the brain stem) that project to the basal ganglia.

Essential Revision Notes for MRCP, 2nd edn, p 553

9. A: Angiotensin I

Angiotensin-converting enzyme (ACE) is a membrane-bound glycoprotein found mostly in the lung that converts angiotensin I to angiotensin II. It also inactivates bradykinin.

10. D: Anion gap

Diabetic ketoacidosis is associated with reduced plasma pH and an elevated anion gap, reflecting the accumulation of acetoacetate and β-hydroxybutyrate (*see* Clinical Biochemistry and Metabolism, Question 29). The arterial $P\text{CO}_2$ will be low in (partial) compensation for the metabolic acidosis.

11. B: Haloperidol

Drugs that can lead to elevated prolactin levels include dopamine receptor antagonists (eg phenothiazines, risperidone, metoclopramide), dopamine-depleting agents (eg methyldopa or reserpine) and a range of others including cocaine, cimetidine, isoniazid, verapamil and tricyclic antidepressants.

12. E: Grand mal seizure

Cerebral blood flow (CBF) is closely coupled to cerebral metabolism in the healthy adult brain. Arterial CO_2 levels are a major determinant of CBF, with increasing $P\text{CO}_2$ associated with enhanced CBF. CBF is also inversely related to haematocrit, decreased by hypothermia. Tachypnoea would be expected to lower arterial $P\text{CO}_2$ and hence lead to either no change or a fall in CBF. However, epileptic seizures stimulate CBF and so this represents the best answer here.

13. C: Positive sharp waves

Denervation leads to a decline in the overall number of motor units activated by movement, but an increase in their firing rate. Chronically, large motor unit potentials of increased duration are seen. Motor conduction times are often normal and motor conduction block does not occur in simple denervation. Fibrillation is a feature of acute denervation and represents random spontaneous firing of individual motor units, together with positive sharp waves and complex repetitive discharges. The F wave is a late response occurring after a compound muscle action potential and reflects anti-dromic stimulation of the anterior horn cells. F waves are often used in the evaluation of neuropathies and plexopathies, but are not useful in denervation.

14. C: Large myelinated nerves

Nerves with greater diameter will conduct faster; also nerves that are myelinated will conduct faster than unmyelinated ones (saltatory conduction).

Essential Revision Notes for MRCP, 2nd edn, p 587

15. A: Flow–volume loop

The shape of the flow–volume curve of a spirometry test can be used to demonstrate different abnormalities of the large central airways, eg intrathoracic, extrathoracic and upper airway obstructions can all be distinguished by their effects on the flow–volume loop. In this case, the goitre would cause a plateau of flow during forced inspiration and forced expiration. FEV_1 and PEFR would also be reduced, although the superior ability of the flow–volume loop to contribute to the differential diagnosis makes this the best answer.

16. B: Hypothermia

The J wave is a hump-like deflection occurring at the junction between the R and ST waves. It is most commonly observed in patients with hypothermia but can also be seen in association with hypercalcaemia, after a head injury or subarachnoid haemorrhage, or during angina.

17. D: Ventilation–perfusion ratio

Alveoli at the lung apex are larger than at the base so they have reduced compliance, resulting in decreased apical ventilation. The apices are also less perfused because they are above the level of the heart, although this reduction is greater than the reduction in ventilation, so that the ventilation–perfusion ratio is overall higher at the apices.

18. C: Arterial pH

Altitude stimulates hyperventilation and a respiratory alkalosis, which then resolves with increased renal excretion of bicarbonate. Hypoxaemia stimulates production of erythropoietin and a resulting increase in red cell mass, plus production of 2,3-DPG (*see* Question 1) shifts the oxygen dissociation curve to the right.

Essential Revision Notes for MRCP, 2nd edn, p 649

19. B: Schilling's test

Schilling's test is used to assess the absorption of vitamin B_{12}. The patient is injected intramuscularly with vitamin B_{12} sufficient to saturate the body stores, and then administered oral vitamin B_{12} radiolabelled with cobalt-58 plus additional vitamin B_{12} radiolabelled with cobalt-57 bound to intrinsic factor. Rapid absorption and excretion (in the urine) should result, with malabsorption indicated by low excretion, and malabsorption specifically caused by pernicious anaemia indicated by an elevated cobalt-57:cobalt-58 ratio.

20. D: Pulsus paradoxus

Cardiac tamponade results from an accumulation of fluid or blood in the pericardium, leading to limited ventricular filling, reduced cardiac output and elevated right-sided cardiac pressures. Thus the jugular venous pressure (JVP) is elevated; there is tachycardia and systolic hypotension, and diminished heart sounds. Pulsus paradoxus is an inspiratory decrease in arterial pressure and is one of the signs of tamponade, although it is not specific and can be seen in other pericardial and pulmonary conditions.

Essential Revision Notes for MRCP, 2nd edn, p 51

21. D: Nitric oxide

Nitric oxide is synthesised in vascular endothelium (it was previously known as endothelium-derived relaxant factor) as well as in other cell types, and is an important modulator of vasodilator tone associated with the regulation of systemic blood pressure.

Essential Revision Notes for MRCP, 2nd edn, p 445

22. D: Hypotension

Renin release from the juxtaglomerular apparatus of the kidney is associated with reduced renal perfusion, β-adrenoceptor stimulation and low sodium delivery. It converts angiotensinogen to angiotensin I as part of a response designed to restore circulating blood volume.

Essential Revision Notes for MRCP, 2nd edn, p 125

23. A: Eisenmenger syndrome

Eisenmenger syndrome results from the reversal of a previous left-to-right cardiac shunt caused by massive pulmonary hypertension. It can therefore result from ventricular septal defect (VSD), ASD or PDA, and leads to central cyanosis.

Essential Revision Notes for MRCP, 2nd edn, p 26

24. E: Gastrin

Gastrin is produced and secreted by G cells located in the antral mucosa of the stomach, and activates parietal cells through direct and indirect mechanisms to release hydrochloric acid.

Essential Revision Notes for MRCP, 2nd edn, p 178

25. D: Tachycardia

The Valsalva manoeuvre is forced expiration against a closed glottis and can be used to assess autonomic control of cardiovascular function. Attempted expiration causes a rise in intrathoracic pressure, resulting in aortic compression and a transient rise in blood pressure, which then causes a transient reflex bradycardia. Reduced venous return (resulting from compression of the vena cava) causes a fall in cardiac output and a corresponding fall in blood pressure with tachycardia. After a few seconds, arterial pressure is reduced and heart rate elevated, making Answer D the best option.

26. D: Isovolumetric contraction

The QRS complex represents the time that it takes for the ventricles to depolarise. The initial negative Q wave reflects electrical activity in the anteroseptal region, with the R wave reflecting the point when roughly half the ventricular myocardium has been depolarised. The QRS complex precedes ventricular ejection, which begins about half-way through the complex and continues to the T wave. The best answer for this question is therefore Answer D, the period of isovolumetric contraction.

27. A: Prolonged P–R interval

Hyperkalaemia can cause tall T waves, a prolonged P–R interval and flattened or absent P waves. In contrast, ST depression, flat or inverted T waves and a prolonged P–R interval are all features of hypokalaemia.

Essential Revision Notes for MRCP, 2nd edn, p 6

28. C: Increased TBG

In normal pregnancy T_3, T_4 and TBG are all increased in concentration, whereas TSH falls in the first or second trimesters, and then rises in the third trimester. The ratio free T_3:T_3 falls in the third trimester.

Essential Revision Notes for MRCP, 2nd edn, p 372

29. D: Decreased sympathetic activity

Renin release from the juxtaglomerular apparatus of the kidney is associated with reduced renal perfusion, β-adrenoceptor stimulation and low sodium delivery. *See also* Question 22.

30. E: Increased osteoclast activity

Release of calcium (and phosphate) from bone is stimulated by increased parathyroid hormone (PTH) and vitamin D. PTH stimulates osteoclastic bone resorption indirectly, as well as stimulating bone formation, renal tubular reabsorption of calcium and renal production of 1,25-dihydroxyvitamin D, to increase calcium absorption from the intestine.

Essential Revision Notes for MRCP, 2nd edn, p 406

31. A: Increased TNF-α

TNF-α is a pro-inflammatory cytokine with a wide range of actions. It is produced by macrophages, eosinophils and natural killer (NK) cells and stimulates prostaglandin production; in addition it induces granulocyte–macrophage colony-stimulating factor (GM-CSF). TNF levels increase in heart failure and predict mortality.

Essential Revision Notes for MRCP, 2nd edn, p 448

32. A: VIP

Gastric acid secretion is enhanced by vagal nerve stimulation, gastrin and histamine but inhibited by somatostatin, VIP, glucagon, secretin, prostaglandin E_2 (PGE_2) and gastric inhibitory polypeptide (GIP). Gastrin and cholecystokinin have overlapping biological effects because they share five C-terminal amino acids, and the gastrin receptor also binds cholecystokinin.

33. D: Increased affinity of haemoglobin for oxygen

Carbon monoxide poisoning results from combination of some of the haemoglobin with carbon monoxide. This gives rise to a decreased arterial concentration of oxygen, but neither affects the partial pressure of oxygen (compare anaemia) or the partial pressure of carbon dioxide. The haemoglobin–oxygen dissociation curve is shifted to the left, reflecting increased affinity of oxygen for haemoglobin, which impedes tissue unloading of oxygen.

Essential Revision Notes for MRCP, 2nd edn, p 90

34. B: Increased pulmonary compliance

Emphysema is characterised by abnormal, permanent enlargement of the air spaces distal to the terminal bronchioles. There is loss of elastic recoil with consequent increased pulmonary compliance and decreased diffusivity, resulting in a decreased FEV_1 and decreased gas transfer factor.

Essential Revision Notes for MRCP, 2nd edn, p 644–6

35. C: Hypernatraemia

Renin is released from the juxtaglomerular apparatus of the kidney in response to reduced delivery of sodium or reduced renal perfusion. Renin is an enzyme responsible for converting angiotensinogen to angiotensin I.

Essential Revision Notes for MRCP, 2nd edn, p 126

36. C: Urinary albumin

Most guidelines recommend measurement of albumin in a spot urine sample as the first step in the screening process for diabetic nephropathy, which should be a routine procedure in patients with diabetes.

37. D: Increased renal blood flow

ANP is synthesised and released by cardiac muscle cells in response to atrial distension, increased angiotensin II levels and sympathetic stimulation. Elevated levels of ANP are found in congestive heart failure. ANP decreases aldosterone release, increases renal blood flow and the glomerular filtration rate (GFR), leads to increased excretion of sodium and decreases release of renin and angiotensin II. The effects of ANP therefore tend to counteract the renin–angiotensin system.

Essential Revision Notes for MRCP, 2nd edn, p 127

38. C: Increased renal blood flow

Blood volume increases progressively in pregnancy, with increased red cell mass. Cardiac output increases, with increased renal and hepatic blood flow. There is a steady reduction in total peripheral resistance over time.

Essential Revision Notes for MRCP, 2nd edn, p 366

39. E: Hypoparathyroidism

Hyperphosphataemia is found most often in association with renal insufficiency but is typically caused by decreased glomerular filtration rather than changes in tubular reabsorption. Tumour lysis syndrome and rhabdomyolysis cause hyperphosphataemia through acutely increasing the serum phosphate load. Hypoparathyroidism increases tubular reabsorption of phosphate, leading to hyperphosphataemia.

Essential Revision Notes for MRCP, 2nd edn, p 417

40. A: Decreased heart rate

Activation of sympathetic efferents to the heart increases heart rate, contractility and conduction velocity. Parasympathetic effects are opposite. In blood vessels, sympathetic activation constricts arteries and arterioles, and in veins it decreases venous blood volume and increases venous pressure. In contrast, most blood vessels do not have parasympathetic innervation.

41. D: Severe hypercapnia without significant hypoxia

Non-invasive ventilation requires an alert, cooperative patient who is able to protect the airway. Although useful in mild hypoxia, it is likely to be more effective in situations characterised by acute hypercapnic respiratory failure.

42. A: Elevated serum troponin

Hypoxia is often seen after pulmonary embolism, with $P\text{CO}_2$ often normal or decreased as a result of tachypnoea. D-dimer is a fibrin degradation product produced by plasmin-mediated proteolysis and is usually elevated in pulmonary embolism, but the test is neither sensitive nor specific enough to be useful diagnostically. Lactate levels are often elevated. Troponin levels are usually elevated after a pulmonary embolism and confer a significantly poorer prognosis.

43. E: Independent P-wave activity

Differentiating broad complex tachycardia of ventricular and supraventricular origin is a classic ECG question. Age (> 35 years) and a previous history of ischaemic heart disease are both strongly predictive of ventricular tachycardia. Direct evidence of independent P-wave activity or the presence of capture or fusion beats is highly suggestive of ventricular tachycardia. QRS complex duration of > 140 ms indicates a ventricular origin, as does concordance through the chest leads.

44. C: Sarcoidosis

Reduction in the FVC with a normal or elevated FEV_1:FVC ratio defines restrictive lung disease spirometrically. In comparison, obstructive lung disease causes disproportionate reduction in the FEV_1 compared with the FVC. Restrictive lung disease can be caused by either diseases intrinsic to lung tissue, thus also affecting transfer factor, or extrinsic disease of the chest wall or pleura.

Essential Revision Notes for MRCP, 2nd edn, p 644

45. B: Conjugated bilirubin

Post-hepatic (obstructive) jaundice is associated with impaired excretion of bile from the liver into the gut. Conjugated bilirubin is reabsorbed, resulting in increased serum and urine levels (and dark urine, with pale stools caused by lack of stercobilinogen). Both transaminases and ALP are elevated, the latter particularly so in obstructive jaundice.

Essential Revision Notes for MRCP, 2nd edn, p 212

46. A: Negative intrathoracic pressure

Diaphragmatic excursion is about one centimetre in normal breathing. Inspiration is associated with a fall in the diaphragm and generation of negative intrathoracic pressure. On expiration the abdominal musculature contracts together with the elastic recoil of the rib cage.

47. E: Vitamin K

This clinical scenario depicts malabsorption of vitamin K, leading to hypoprothrombinaemia with easy bruising and a bleeding tendency. Vitamin K is a fat-soluble vitamin and a variety of gastrointestinal diseases can cause malabsorption, eg coeliac sprue, Crohn's disease, ulcerative colitis and chronic pancreatitis.

48. C: Cardiac output falls

Mechanical ventilation causes a decrease in cardiac output through the increased intrathoracic pressure, leading to decreased venous return. Increased intrathoracic pressure also leads to decreased intrathoracic blood volume and the increased lung volumes result in a rise in pulmonary vascular resistance.

Chapter 5
GENETICS
Questions

---

1. Which one of the following is most likely to be a feature of Turner syndrome?

- ☐ A Horseshoe kidney
- ☐ B Ovarian agenesis
- ☐ C Aortic coarctation
- ☐ D Uterine agenesis
- ☐ E Adrenal hypoplasia

2. Which one of the following disorders is polygenic?

- ☐ A Ankylosing spondylitis
- ☐ B Huntington's disease
- ☐ C Down syndrome
- ☐ D Fragile X
- ☐ E Erythropoietic protoporphyria

Answers on pages 123–132

3. A 43-year-old woman presents with irregular jerking of her arms and legs. Her husband reports that recently she is 'fidgety' and has poor concentration. What is genetic testing most likely to show?

- ☐ A Trisomy
- ☐ B Point mutations or deletions
- ☐ C Trinucleotide repeat expansion
- ☐ D Monosomy
- ☐ E Additional X chromosome

4. Which one of the following disorders is inherited through mitochondrial DNA mutations?

- ☐ A Holt–Oram syndrome
- ☐ B Parkinson's disease
- ☐ C Leber's optic atrophy
- ☐ D Prader–Willi syndrome
- ☐ E von Willebrand's disease

5. Which one of the following diseases is a chromosomal disorder?

- ☐ A Duchenne muscular dystrophy
- ☐ B Refsum's disease
- ☐ C Spinocerebellar ataxia
- ☐ D Klinefelter syndrome
- ☐ E Cystic fibrosis

6. What is the most appropriate laboratory technique for diagnosing chromosomal trisomy?

- ☐ A Karyotyping
- ☐ B Immunohistochemistry
- ☐ C Polymerase chain reaction (PCR)
- ☐ D Gene sequencing
- ☐ E Southern blotting

7. A 54-year-old woman presents with primary hyperparathyroidism some years after treatment for a prolactinoma. What is the most likely diagnosis?

- ☐ A Neurofibromatosis
- ☐ B Multiple endocrine neoplasia type 1 (MEN1)
- ☐ C Familial parathyroid hyperplasia
- ☐ D von Hippel–Lindau syndrome
- ☐ E Familial paraganglionoma

8. Which one of the following disorders is inherited in an autosomal recessive fashion?

- ☐ A Achondroplasia
- ☐ B Glucose 6-phosphate dehydrogenase (G6PD) deficiency
- ☐ C Huntington's disease
- ☐ D Wilson's disease
- ☐ E Ehlers–Danlos syndrome

9. Which one of the following disorders is inherited in an autosomal dominant fashion?

- ☐ A Ataxia–telangiectasia
- ☐ B Neurofibromatosis type 1
- ☐ C Homocystinuria
- ☐ D Gilbert syndrome
- ☐ E Fabry's disease

10. Which one of the following disorders is inherited in a polygenic fashion?

- ☐ A Friedreich's ataxia
- ☐ B Fragile X syndrome
- ☐ C Huntington's disease
- ☐ D Bipolar (manic–depressive) disorder
- ☐ E Cystic fibrosis

11. Which one of the following genetic disorders confers an increased risk of cancer?

- ☐ A Niemann–Pick disease
- ☐ B Ataxia–telangiectasia
- ☐ C Cystic fibrosis
- ☐ D Duchenne muscular dystrophy
- ☐ E Haemophilia A

12. Mutation of which one of the following genes is likely to be the most important genetic risk factor for breast cancer?

☐ A *p53*

☐ B *ATM*

☐ C *BRCA*-1

☐ D *APOE*

☐ E *HER2/neu*

13. Which one of the following conditions is most likely to predispose to the development of breast cancer?

☐ A Goodpasture syndrome

☐ B Down syndrome

☐ C Chédiak–Higashi syndrome

☐ D von Hippel–Lindau syndrome

☐ E Ataxia–telangiectasia

14. Which one of the following disorders is caused by expansion of a trinucleotide repeat sequence?

☐ A Noonan syndrome

☐ B Fragile X syndrome

☐ C Fanconi's anaemia

☐ D Spinal muscular atrophy

☐ E Fabry's disease

Answers on pages 123–132

15. Which one of the following terms is most appropriate for a mutation that changes a codon from one amino acid to another?

☐ A Frameshift

☐ B Nonsense

☐ C Silent

☐ D Missense

☐ E Point

16. Which one of the following is most likely to be a feature of mitochondrial genetic disease?

☐ A Higher prevalence in females than in males

☐ B Higher prevalence in males than in females

☐ C Only transmitted maternally

☐ D Transmitted both maternally and paternally

☐ E Only transmitted paternally

17. Which one of the following factors is most likely to be deficient in classic haemophilia?

☐ A Factor VIII

☐ B Factor IX

☐ C Factor III

☐ D Factor V

☐ E Factor VI

18. What are contiguous regulatory regions of a gene that control gene expression known as?

- ☐ A Exons
- ☐ B Transcription factors
- ☐ C Enhancers
- ☐ D Introns
- ☐ E Promoters

19. Neurofibromatosis type I is associated with point mutations on which chromosome?

- ☐ A Chromosome 16
- ☐ B Chromosome 19
- ☐ C Chromosome 5
- ☐ D Chromosome 22
- ☐ E Chromosome 17

20. A chromosomal abnormality is characteristic of which one of the following disorders?

- ☐ A Marfan syndrome
- ☐ B Edwards syndrome
- ☐ C Achondroplasia
- ☐ D Neurofibromatosis
- ☐ E Fragile X syndrome

Answers on pages 123–132

21. Which one of the following methods can be used to generate large amounts of DNA from small samples?

☐ A Comparative genomic hybridisation (CGH)

☐ B Southern blotting

☐ C Fluorescent *in situ* hybridisation (FISH)

☐ D Flow sorting

☐ E Polymerase chain reaction (PCR)

22. Genetic variation in which one of the following genes is most likely to increase the risk of developing Alzheimer's disease?

☐ A *ATP7B*

☐ B *ATM*

☐ C *BRCA*-1

☐ D Transferrin

☐ E Apolipoprotein E (*APOE*) gene

23. Which one of the following terms may explain why a genetic disease gets worse as the patient gets older?

☐ A Somatic instability

☐ B Anticipation

☐ C Variable penetrance

☐ D Lyonisation

☐ E Opsonisation

24. Which one of the following phenotypes is most likely to be associated with mutations of mitochondrial DNA?

- ☐ A Stroke in a young person
- ☐ B Epilepsy
- ☐ C Prion disease
- ☐ D Ataxia
- ☐ E Chorea

25. A woman with cystic fibrosis has a husband who is heterozygous for the cystic fibrosis mutation. What is the likelihood that their children may have cystic fibrosis?

- ☐ A 0%
- ☐ B 25%
- ☐ C 50%
- ☐ D 75%
- ☐ E 100%

26. A woman who is heterozygous for an X-linked recessive condition marries an asymptomatic man. Which one of the following statements is most likely to be correct?

- ☐ A Half their male offspring will have the condition
- ☐ B Half their male offspring will be carriers
- ☐ C Half their female offspring will have the condition
- ☐ D Half their offspring will have the condition
- ☐ E None of their female offspring will be carriers

Answers on pages 123–132

27. Which one of the following genetic disorders is most likely to be associated with short stature?

- ☐ A Klinefelter syndrome
- ☐ B Marfan syndrome
- ☐ C Edwards syndrome
- ☐ D Fragile X syndrome
- ☐ E Turner syndrome

28. Metabolism of which one of the following drugs is most likely to be determined genetically?

- ☐ A Amoxicillin
- ☐ B Isoniazid
- ☐ C Phenytoin
- ☐ D Xylocaine
- ☐ E Ciprofloxacin

29. Which one of the following statements about the children of a female carrier of an X-linked recessive disease is correct?

- ☐ A Half her sons will have the disease
- ☐ B Half her daughters will have the disease
- ☐ C Half her children will have the disease
- ☐ D None of her daughters will be carriers
- ☐ E Half her sons will be carriers

30. What is the most common human leucocyte-associated antigen (HLA) type in rheumatoid arthritis?

☐ A HLA-B12

☐ B HLA-B27

☐ C HLA-DP

☐ D HLA-DR2

☐ E HLA-DR4

31. Mutations in which one of the following genes account for most cases of familial breast cancer?

☐ A *BRCA*-1

☐ B *p53*

☐ C *PTEN*

☐ D *ATM*

☐ E *p65*

32. A man with common variable immunodeficiency would like to start a family. Approximately what percentage of his children are most likely to inherit his disease?

☐ A 0%

☐ B 25%

☐ C 50%

☐ D 75%

☐ E 100%

Answers on pages 123–132

33. A 32-year-old non-smoker presents with emphysema and has abnormal liver function tests; a liver biopsy reveals cirrhosis. What is the most likely genotype for this genetic disorder?

- ☐ A *PiMM*
- ☐ B *PiMZ*
- ☐ C *PiSZ*
- ☐ D *PiZZ*
- ☐ E *PiSS*

34. What is the approximate lifetime risk of developing type 1 diabetes mellitus for an asymptomatic young woman whose identical twin has recently been diagnosed with this disorder?

- ☐ A 2%
- ☐ B 5%
- ☐ C 25%
- ☐ D 50%
- ☐ E 100%

35. A young man with learning disabilities is tall with sparse secondary sexual characteristics, enlarged breasts, and small testicles and penis. What is the most likely karyotype?

- ☐ A 47,XYY
- ☐ B 47,XXY
- ☐ C 46,XY
- ☐ D 46,XO
- ☐ E 45,XO

36. A 45-year-old man complaining of tiredness is found to have the following full blood count (FBC):

Haemoglobin (Hb)	9.0 g/dl
White blood cell count (WCC)	105 x 10/l
Platelets	600 x 10^9/l

Which one of the following chromosomal abnormalities (translocations) is most likely to be associated with these findings?

- ☐ A t(9,13)
- ☐ B t(3,13)
- ☐ C t(9,22)
- ☐ D t(21,22)
- ☐ E t(6,9)

GENETICS
Answers

1. **B: Ovarian agenesis**

Individuals with Turner syndrome have the karyotype 45,X and ovarian agenesis is the cardinal feature. Phenotypically, individuals with Turner syndrome have a webbed or short neck, low hairline and widely spaced nipples. Renal abnormalities are seen in about 30% and cardiovascular anomalies (eg coarctation) in between 10–35%.

Essential Revision Notes for MRCP, 2nd edn, p 232

2. **A: Ankylosing spondylitis**

Huntington's disease and fragile X syndrome are both trinucleotide repeat disorders; Down syndrome results from trisomy 21 and erythropoietic protoporphyria arises from a mutation of the ferrochelatase gene (chromosome 18).

3. **C: Trinucleotide repeat expansion**

This history is most consistent with Huntington's disease, a trinucleotide repeat disorder inherited as an autosomal dominant. There is variable expansion of a CAG trinucleotide repeat in the huntingtin (HD) gene on chromosome 4.

Essential Revision Notes for MRCP, 2nd edn, pp 238, 554–5

4. C: Leber's optic atrophy

Mitochondrial DNA (mtDNA) is maternally inherited and mutates much more frequently than nuclear DNA. Leber's optic atrophy is a mitochondrially inherited acute or subacute loss of central vision predominantly affecting young men.

Essential Revision Notes for MRCP, 2nd edn, p 457

5. D: Klinefelter syndrome

A chromosomal disorder is one that affects a whole chromosome or chromosome segment and is distinct from single gene disorders. Down syndrome is the most common chromosomal disorder. In the list of options given, Klinefelter syndrome (47 XXY) is the only chromosomal disorder.

6. A: Karyotyping

Karyotyping is a procedure to identify macroscopic chromosomal abnormalities by counting the number of chromosomes and identifying large-scale structural changes. Chromosomal disorders (*see* Question 5) such as Down syndrome can be diagnosed in this way. In comparison, the other techniques amplify fragments of DNA (PCR), look at individual genes (gene sequencing), identify specific sequences of DNA (Southern blotting) or detect antigens in tissue using antibodies (immunohistochemistry).

7. B: MEN1

The combination of parathyroid tumours, pituitary hyperplasia or tumour and pancreatic islet cell tumours is known as MEN1. Hyperparathyroidism is the most common manifestation, and prolactinomas are the most common pituitary tumour in patients with MEN1. Peak incidence is in the third decade for women and the fourth decade for men, with women being affected more frequently.

Essential Revision Notes for MRCP, 2nd edn, p 144

8. D: Wilson's disease

Achondroplasia is the most common type of short-limbed dwarfism and is inherited as an autosomal dominant through mutations in the *FGFR3* gene. G6PD deficiency is an X-linked recessive disorder. Huntington's disease is caused by trinucleotide repeat expansion in the *HD* gene, inherited as an autosomal dominant disorder. Ehlers–Danlos syndromes are caused by a variety of mutations in several genes but are all autosomal dominant. Finally, Wilson's disease is an autosomal recessive disorder caused by mutations in the *ATP7B* gene.

9. B: Neurofibromatosis type 1

Ataxia–telangiectasia is caused by mutations in the *ATM* gene and inherited in an autosomal recessive fashion. Homocystinuria is also an autosomal recessive disorder with various gene defects. Fabry's disease is X-linked recessive and caused by mutations in the *GLA* gene. Gilbert syndrome is the most common inherited cause of unconjugated hyperbilirubinaemia and is an autosomal recessive condition. Neurofibromatosis type 1 is caused by mutations in the *NF1* gene and has autosomal dominant inheritance.

10. D: Bipolar disorder

Friedreich's ataxia is an autosomal recessive trinucleotide repeat disease, whereas fragile X syndrome and Huntington's disease are autosomal dominant trinucleotide repeat disorders. Cystic fibrosis is a monogenic autosomal recessive disorder. Inheritance patterns of bipolar disorder are complex but considered to be polygenic.

11. B: Ataxia–telangiectasia

Ataxia–telangiectasia is caused by mutations in the *ATM* gene and is inherited in an autosomal recessive pattern. The *ATM* gene product plays an important role in controlling cell division and DNA repair, and so mutations in the gene can prevent cells from responding correctly to DNA damage, or induce premature apoptosis. At least 10% of patients will develop cancer, particularly lymphoma or leukaemia.

12. C: *BRCA*-1

BRCA-1 and *BRCA*-2 are the most common genes related to hereditary breast cancer. Mutations in these genes (which are tumour-suppressor genes) give a very high lifetime risk of developing breast cancer. *BRCA*-1 mutations also increase the risk of ovarian and colon cancers (and prostate cancer in men). Mutations in *BRCA*-1 and *BRCA*-2 are inherited in an autosomal dominant pattern. *ATM* and *HER2/neu* (*ERBB2*) mutations also increase risk, but not by as much.

13. E: Ataxia–telangiectasia

See answers to Questions 11 and 12.

14. B: Fragile X syndrome

The genetic mutation in trinucleotide repeat disorders is a repetitive sequence of three nucleotides that can undergo expansion. Examples of trinucleotide repeat disorders include Huntington's disease, Fragile X syndrome, myotonic dystrophy, Friedreich's ataxia and spinocerebellar ataxias.

15. D: Missense

A frameshift mutation occurs when the addition or loss of DNA bases changes the reading frame (each codon or group of three bases that code for one amino acid) of a gene. A nonsense mutation is a change in one DNA base-pair that prematurely stops protein synthesis. A silent mutation is one in which the function of the protein product of the gene remains unchanged. A missense mutation is a change in one DNA base-pair in a codon, which results in the substitution of one amino acid for another in the gene product. A 'point mutation' is a general term for any alteration in the DNA sequence caused by a single nucleotide base change, insertion or deletion.

16. C: Only transmitted maternally

Mitochondria contain their own distinct genome and mutations in this genome are responsible for specific syndromes that are maternally inherited, because ova contain mitochondria whereas sperm do not.

Essential Revision Notes for MRCP, 2nd edn, p 457

17. A: Factor VIII

Haemophilia A ('classic' haemophilia) is the most common form of this disease, inherited in an X-linked recessive fashion and caused by mutations in the *F8* gene. This gene encodes coagulation factor VIII. Mutations in the *F9* gene (encoding coagulation factor IX) cause the rarer haemophilia B ('Christmas disease').

18. E: Promoters

The promoter region is just upstream from a gene and acts as a binding site for transcription factors and RNA polymerase during initiation of transcription. In contrast, introns are non-coding and exons code portions of genes.

19. E: Chromosome 17

Neurofibromatosis type 1 is caused by mutations in the *NF1* gene on chromosome 17 and is inherited as an autosomal dominant disorder. Clinically, neurofibromas grow along nerves in the skin, brain and other parts of the body. Cancer, including cerebral tumours and leukaemia, can occur in about 10% of patients.

20. B: Edwards syndrome

Edwards syndrome is caused by trisomy 18, and is the only disorder from the possible options caused by an abnormality in the number of chromosomes. Changes in chromosome structure can also cause chromosomal disorders.

21. E: PCR

PCR is an amplification reaction where small amounts of target DNA (known as the 'template') are amplified to produce a much larger amount of DNA sufficient to undergo more detailed analyses.

22. E: *APOE* gene

About three-quarters of Alzheimer's disease is sporadic and the remaining quarter hereditary, caused by mutations in the amyloid precursor protein (*APP*), presenilin 1 (*PSEN1*) or presenilin 2 (*PSEN2*) genes. Variability in the *APOE* gene increases the overall risk of developing Alzheimer's disease, In particular, the presence of the ε4 allele of *APOE* increases the chances of developing the disease in a dose-dependent fashion (with two ε4 alleles conferring greater risk than a single allele). The *ATP7B* gene is mutated in Wilson's disease and *ATM* in ataxia–telangiectasia, and *BRCA*-1 mutations confer increased risk of breast cancer.

23. A: Somatic instability

Somatic instability can occur in trinucleotide repeat disorders where the length of the expansion (*See* Question 14) increases over time as cells divide throughout the life of the individual. This may explain why some trinucleotide disorders, such as myotonic dystrophy, get worse as the individual gets older.

24. A: Stroke in a young person

Neurological phenotypes associated with mtDNA mutations include sensorineural deafness, optic atrophy, pigmentary retinopathy, stroke in young people and myopathy. *See also* Question 16.

Essential Revision Notes for MRCP, 2nd edn, p 457

25. C: 50%

When both parents are carriers (heterozygous) for an autosomal recessive trait, there is a 25% chance of a child inheriting abnormal genes from both parents and therefore of developing the disease. However, in this case the mother is already homozygous for the abnormal gene and so the chance of their children inheriting abnormal genes from both parents is 50% because the husband is heterozygous. Note that although cystic fibrosis is associated with fertility problems in men (95% are infertile), only 20% of women with cystic fibrosis are infertile.

26. A: Half their male offspring will have the condition

Women are usually unaffected by X-linked recessive conditions (although they may have mild manifestations as a result of lyonisation). Sons of a female carrier have a 50% chance of being affected and daughters have a 50% chance of being carriers.

Essential Revision Notes for MRCP, 2nd edn, p 237

27. E: Turner syndrome

Turner syndrome is a chromosomal disorder of females characterised by short stature and lack of sexual development, and caused by complete or partial absence of one X chromosome.
Essential Revision Notes for MRCP, 2nd edn, p 232

28. B: Isoniazid

Hydralazine, procainamide, phenelzine, dapsone, some sulphonamides.

29. A: Half her sons will have the disease

Women are usually unaffected by X-linked recessive conditions (although they may have mild manifestations as a result of lyonisation). Sons of a female carrier have a 50% chance of being affected and daughters a 50% chance of being carriers. *See* Question 26.

Essential Revision Notes for MRCP, 2nd edn, p 237

30. E: HLA-DR4

Genetic factors account for about 10–30% of the risk of developing rheumatoid arthritis, which has a specific association with HLA-DR4. Patients with HLA-DR4 have a worse prognosis.
Essential Revision Notes for MRCP, 2nd edn, pp 320, 696

31. A: *BRCA*-1

BRCA-1 and *BRCA*-2 are the most common genes related to hereditary breast cancer. *See* Question and answer 12.

32. A: 0%

Common variable immunodeficiency is the most prevalent primary immunodeficiency and is characterised by low levels of most or all immunoglobulins, deficiency of B lymphocytes and consequent recurrent bacterial infections. It is diverse in both clinical presentation and underlying deficits. There is some evidence that genetic factors are involved, eg about 20% of patients will have a selective IgA deficiency. However, it has no clear pattern of inheritance and most patients are sporadic cases with no family history.

Essential Revision Notes for MRCP, 2nd edn, p 330

33. D: *PiZZ*

Emphysema in an individual under the age of 40 suggests α_1-antitrypsin deficiency, particularly in associated with liver cirrhosis. The *SERPINA*-1 gene for α_1-antitrypsin is on chromosome 14 and expressed in hepatocytes and mononuclear phagocytes. The disorder is inherited in an autosomal co-dominant pattern, meaning that two different versions of the gene may be expressed. The most common version of the allele, *M*, results in normal levels of α_1-antitrypsin. *S* and *Z* alleles produce moderate or very low levels of the protein. The most severe genotype – *PiZZ* – causes the most severe manifestations of emphysema and cirrhosis, as here.

Essential Revision Notes for MRCP, 2nd edn, pp 654–5

34. D: 50%

Concordance rates for type 1 (insulin-dependent) diabetes are higher in monozygotic than in dizygotic twins, and reach up to 50–60% lifetime risk for monozygotic twins, compared with less than 10% for dizygotic twins.

Essential Revision Notes for MRCP, 2nd edn, p 149

35. B: 47,XXY

The phenotype described is consistent with Klinefelter syndrome, which is found in about 1 in every 500–1000 newborn males and is associated with the karyotypic presence of an extra copy of chromosome-X. Semen count and serum testosterone are low whereas serum oestradiol, luteinising hormone (LH) and follicle-stimulating hormone (FSH) are high. Testosterone therapy is often used. Learning disabilities are common.

Essential Revision Notes for MRCP, 2nd edn, p 232

36. C: t(9,22)

Of cases with chronic myeloid leukaemia (CML) 90% have a balanced translocation between chromosomes 9 and 22, termed t(9,22). This is known as the Philadelphia chromosome with the breakpoints at the *BCR* gene on chromosome 22 and the *ABL* gene on chromosome 9. CML presents in middle age with tiredness, weight loss and sweating and is associated with high white cell counts (100–500 x 10^9/l).

Chapter 6

IMMUNOLOGY

Questions

---

1. Which one of the following HLA antigens is most commonly associated with narcolepsy?

☐ A HLA-DR2

☐ B HLA-Dw3

☐ C HLA-B14

☐ D HLA-B27

☐ E HLA-A3

2. A 23-year-old man is found to have low serum C3 with normal serum C4 concentration. Which one of the following is the most likely underlying diagnosis?

☐ A Mesangiocapillary glomerulonephritis

☐ B Anaphylaxis

☐ C Hereditary C1 esterase inhibitor deficiency

☐ D Rheumatoid arthritis

☐ E Systemic lupus erythematosus (SLE) nephritis

Answers on pages 151–163

3. What is the most important function of interleukin-2 (IL-2) in the immune response?

- ☐ A Activates complement
- ☐ B Stimulates CD4-cell production
- ☐ C Stimulates B-cell proliferation
- ☐ D Required for antigen presentation
- ☐ E Inhibits clotting

4. Which one of the following statements about secretory IgA is most likely to be correct?

- ☐ A Transferred across the placenta to the fetus
- ☐ B Activates complement by the classic pathway
- ☐ C Responsible for mucosal immunity
- ☐ D Consists of four discrete subclasses
- ☐ E Is assembled in lymph nodes

5. Which one of the following is most important as a cause of renal scarring in glomerulonephritis?

- ☐ A TGF-β (transforming growth factor β)
- ☐ B IL-2
- ☐ C IL-1
- ☐ D PDGF (platelet-derived growth factor)
- ☐ E Nitric oxide (NO)

6. In which one of the following disorders is a positive titre of cytoplasmic anti-neutrophil cytoplasmic antibodies most likely?

- ☐ A Wegener's granulomatosis
- ☐ B Silicosis
- ☐ C Giant cell arteritis
- ☐ D Sarcoidosis
- ☐ E Polyarteritis nodosa

7. Which one of the following disorders is most likely to be associated with a type IV hypersensitivity reaction?

- ☐ A Asthma
- ☐ B Graves' disease
- ☐ C Pulmonary aspergillosis
- ☐ D Sarcoidosis
- ☐ E Goodpasture syndrome

8. A 32-year-old woman with SLE is reviewed in the obstetric clinic at 20 weeks' gestation. The fetal heart rate is 50/min and fetal ECG reveals complete heart block. Which antibody is most likely to be responsible?

- ☐ A Anti-RNP
- ☐ B Anti-La
- ☐ C Anti-Sm
- ☐ D Anti-Jo
- ☐ E Anti-Ro

Answers on pages 151–163

9. Which one of the following laboratory findings is most consistent with a diagnosis of primary biliary cirrhosis?

- ☐ A Anti-double-stranded DNA (dsDNA) antibodies
- ☐ B c-ANCA
- ☐ C p-ANCA
- ☐ D Anti-smooth muscle antibodies
- ☐ E Anti-mitochondrial antibodies

10. Which one of the following vaccines should be avoided in an immunocompromised patient?

- ☐ A Varicella
- ☐ B Diphtheria
- ☐ C Hepatitis B
- ☐ D BCG (bacille Calmette Guérin)
- ☐ E Tetanus

11. The presence of which one of the following autoantibodies would be most supportive of a diagnosis of systemic sclerosis?

- ☐ A SCL-70
- ☐ B Ro
- ☐ C Histone
- ☐ D Jo
- ☐ E Centromere

12. A 46-year-old presents with diplopia and difficulty chewing and swallowing, which grows worse through the day. Which one of the following immunological abnormalities is most likely to be present?

☐ A Anti-thymus antibodies

☐ B Anti-striated muscle antibodies

☐ C Anti-smooth muscle antibodies

☐ D Anti-edrophonium antibodies

☐ E Anti-acetylcholine receptor antibodies

13. For which one of the following does the pathogenic antibody in Graves' disease have specificity?

☐ A Thyroglobulin

☐ B TRH (thyrotrophin-releasing hormone)

☐ C TRH receptors

☐ D TSH (thyroid-stimulating hormone)

☐ E TSH receptors

14. What type of hypersensitivity reaction is responsible for transfusion reactions?

☐ A Type I

☐ B Type II

☐ C Type III

☐ D Type IV

☐ E Type V

15. Which one of the following vaccines should not be given to a 46-year-old HIV-positive man?

- ☐ A Yellow fever
- ☐ B Hepatitis B
- ☐ C Influenza
- ☐ D Pneumococcus
- ☐ E Cholera

16. Which one of the following cell types is most likely to be used in the production of monoclonal antibodies?

- ☐ A Human B lymphocytes
- ☐ B Human T lymphocytes
- ☐ C Mouse T lymphocytes
- ☐ D Human stem cells
- ☐ E Mouse B lymphocytes

17. Which one of the following antibody classes is most likely to be involved in immediate-type hypersensitivity?

- ☐ A IgD
- ☐ B IgE
- ☐ C IgA
- ☐ D IgG
- ☐ E IgM

18. Which one of the following immunoglobulin types is most likely to be a cause of complement activation by the alternative pathway?

☐ A IgE

☐ B IgD

☐ C IgM

☐ D IgA

☐ E IgG

19. Which one of the following cell types is most likely to be tissue bound?

☐ A Basophils

☐ B Eosinophils

☐ C Mast cells

☐ D Neutrophils

☐ E T lymphocytes

20. Which component of the immune system is most likely to be defective in chronic lymphocytic leukaemia (CLL)?

☐ A Mast cells

☐ B B cells

☐ C Macrophages

☐ D Complement

☐ E Immunoglobulin

Answers on pages 151–163

21. In renal transplantation, compatibility at which HLA locus has the greatest influence on graft outcome?

- ☐ A HLA-DR
- ☐ B HLA-A
- ☐ C HLA-DQ
- ☐ D HLA-C
- ☐ E HLA-DP

22. Which one of the following cell types is the commonest in peripheral blood?

- ☐ A T cells
- ☐ B B cells
- ☐ C Eosinophils
- ☐ D Basophils
- ☐ E Mast cells

23. Which one of the following is a monoclonal antibody used in clinical practice?

- ☐ A Cyclophosphamide
- ☐ B Ifosfamide
- ☐ C Cytarabine
- ☐ D Vincristine
- ☐ E Trastuzumab

24. A 42-year-old man with progressive cognitive decline and periventricular white matter lesions on magnetic resonance imaging (MRI) tests positive for the presence of JC viral DNA in his cerebrospinal fluid (CSF). Which one of the following antibodies is likely to be present on serological testing?

- ☐ A Hepatitis B
- ☐ B HIV
- ☐ C Anti-Hu
- ☐ D Anti-Ro
- ☐ E Prion protein

25. A positive test for cold agglutinins in a 26-year-old with pneumonia is most likely to be associated with which causative organism?

- ☐ A *Pneumocystis carinii*
- ☐ B *Haemophilus influenzae*
- ☐ C *Klebsiella pneumoniae*
- ☐ D *Mycoplasma pneumoniae*
- ☐ E *Aspergillus* species

26. In a patient with abnormal neutrophil function, which one of the following bacteria are most likely to be associated with recurrent infection?

- ☐ A *Staphylococcus aureus*
- ☐ B *Streptococcus pneumoniae*
- ☐ C *Legionella pneumophila*
- ☐ D *Giardia lamblia*
- ☐ E *Streptococcus pyogenes*

Answers on pages 151–163

27. Which one of the following best describes Sézary syndrome?

- ☐ A B-cell malignancy
- ☐ B T-cell malignancy
- ☐ C Macrophage disorder
- ☐ D Neutrophil disorder
- ☐ E Mast cell disorder

28. Which one of the following is a co-receptor for entry of HIV into cells?

- ☐ A CD3
- ☐ B CD4
- ☐ C CD8
- ☐ D MHC class II antigen
- ☐ E MHC class I antigen

29. Which one of the following bacteria is most likely to use antigenic variation to overcome the host immune system?

- ☐ A *Mycoplasma pneumoniae*
- ☐ B *Haemophilus influenzae*
- ☐ C *Streptococcus pyogenes*
- ☐ D *Borrelia recurrentis*
- ☐ E *Staphylococcus aureus*

30. Which one of the following is recognised as an antigen-presenting cell type?

- ☐ A Microglia
- ☐ B Eosinophils
- ☐ C Langerhans' cells
- ☐ D Neutrophils
- ☐ E Mast cells

31. Which one of the following is an effect of tumour necrosis factor α (TNF-α)?

- ☐ A Inhibition of angiogenesis
- ☐ B Inhibition of IL-1 expression
- ☐ C Activation of NF-κB transcription factor
- ☐ D Inhibition of acute phase response
- ☐ E Inhibition of IL-6 expression

32. Which one of the following disorders is most likely to be associated with a very high titre of rheumatoid factor?

- ☐ A Rheumatoid arthritis
- ☐ B Mixed cryoglobulinaemia
- ☐ C Wegener's granulomatosis
- ☐ D Kawasaki's disease
- ☐ E Progressive systemic sclerosis

Answers on pages 151–163

33. What type of hypersensitivity reaction is responsible for graft-versus-host disease?

- ☐ A Type I
- ☐ B Type II
- ☐ C Type III
- ☐ D Type IV
- ☐ E Type V

34. What is the most likely normal function of the cell surface CD4 molecule?

- ☐ A Binds to IL-2
- ☐ B Binds to ICAM-1
- ☐ C MHC class I interaction
- ☐ D MHC class II interaction
- ☐ E HIV cell entry

35. A young boy has his second episode of meningitis caused by *Neisseria*. Which one of the following complement factors is most likely to be deficient?

- ☐ A C1
- ☐ B C2
- ☐ C C3
- ☐ D C4
- ☐ E C5

36. A 28-year-old man presents with haematuria and haemoptysis. Which one of the following investigations is most likely to be helpful in reaching a diagnosis?

☐ A Renal ultrasonography

☐ B Chest computed tomography (CT)

☐ C Renal biopsy

☐ D Serum anti-nuclear antibody (ANA)

☐ E Serum α_1-antitrypsin

37. Which one of the following vasculitides is most likely to affect large vessels?

☐ A Kawasaki's disease

☐ B Wegener's granulomatosis

☐ C Polyarteritis nodosa

☐ D Takayasu's arteritis

☐ E Cryoglobulinaemia

38. Which one of the following cell types is most likely to be involved in antigen presentation?

☐ A Langerhans' cells

☐ B Mast cells

☐ C Basophils

☐ D Neutrophils

☐ E Red blood cells

Answers on pages 151–163

39. A 64-year-old woman presents with dyspepsia and intermittent dysphagia in the context of longstanding fatigue and cold feet. Blood tests show:

ANA positive	1:80
Anti-centromere antibodies	Positive
RNP	Positive
Ro	Negative
La	Negative

What is the most likely diagnosis?

- ☐ A Dermatomyositis
- ☐ B Mixed connective tissue disease
- ☐ C Primary Sjögren syndrome
- ☐ D Limited scleroderma
- ☐ E SLE

40. Which one of the following autoantibodies is most specific for a diagnosis of SLE?

- ☐ A Antibodies to extractable nuclear antigens (ENAs)
- ☐ B Antibodies to dsDNA
- ☐ C Anti-phospholipid antibodies
- ☐ D Anti-neutrophil antibodies
- ☐ E RF

41. Which one of the following is least likely to occur in Sjögren syndrome?

- ☐ A Cardiac fibrosis
- ☐ B Parotid gland enlargement
- ☐ C Renal tubular acidosis
- ☐ D Pancreatitis
- ☐ E Corneal ulceration

42. What constitutes Bence Jones protein found in the urine in myeloma?

- ☐ A Ig molecules
- ☐ B Ig light chains
- ☐ C Cryoglobulins
- ☐ D Ig heavy chains
- ☐ E Albumin

43. A 27-year-old woman with SLE complains of fatigue and is found to have a low Hb level and spherocytosis. Which test is most likely to yield the diagnosis?

- ☐ A Bleeding time
- ☐ B Serum ferritin
- ☐ C Vitamin B_{12} level
- ☐ D Prothrombin time
- ☐ E Direct Coombs' test

Answers on pages 151–163

44. Which one of the following findings is least likely to be consistent with a diagnosis of ankylosing spondylitis?

- ☐ A Absence of HLA-B27
- ☐ B Fusion of sacroiliac joints
- ☐ C Loss of lumbar lordosis
- ☐ D Normal C-reactive protein (CRP)
- ☐ E Normal alkaline phosphatase (ALP)

45. Which one of the following characterises the autoantibodies responsible for myasthenia gravis?

- ☐ A Polyclonal origin
- ☐ B Monoclonal origin
- ☐ C Do not fix complement
- ☐ D IgM subtype
- ☐ E IgA subtype

46. Which one of the following is most likely to be a poor prognostic factor in a patient with rheumatoid arthritis?

- ☐ A Low erythrocyte sedimentation rate (ESR)
- ☐ B High RF titre
- ☐ C Female sex
- ☐ D No family history
- ☐ E Absence of extra-articular features

47. Which one of the following laboratory findings is most consistent with a diagnosis of benign paraproteinaemia?

- ☐ A Lytic spinal lesions
- ☐ B Elevated serum creatinine
- ☐ C Bence Jones proteinuria
- ☐ D Low levels of paraprotein
- ☐ E Depressed levels of non-paraprotein Ig

48. Which one of the following antibodies is most likely to be found in a patient diagnosed with Wegener's granulomatosis?

- ☐ A Anti-dsDNA
- ☐ B c-ANCA
- ☐ C RF
- ☐ D p-ANCA
- ☐ E Anti-Ro

IMMUNOLOGY
Answers

1. B: HLA-Dw3

The HLA (human leucocyte antigen) system (short arm of chromosome 6) consists of a series of closely linked genes, the products of which are primarily concerned with the regulation and mediation of immune reactions. The HLA class I genes (the A, B and C loci) are expressed on most nucleated cells, whereas the class II genes (DP, DQ and DR loci) are expressed on B lymphocytes, activated T cells and macrophages. Possession of the HLA-DR2 subtype confers a 50-fold increased risk of developing narcolepsy (the strongest association between any disease and HLA) for reasons that are currently unknown.

2. A: Mesangiocapillary glomerulonephritis

Complement comprises a group of protease precursors and regulating proteins produced by the liver, and presents in normal serum that can act as a mediator of inflammation. Low C3 reflects activation of either the classic or the alternative pathway. C4 levels will be depressed if used by the classic pathway (eg in SLE and rheumatoid arthritis, or in factor VI inhibitor deficiency). Low C3 with a normal C4 therefore occurs with isolated alternative pathway activation. In mesangiocapillary glomerulonephritis this is a result of production of an autoantibody, C3 nephritic factor, that activates this pathway directly.

3. B: Stimulates CD4-cell production

IL-2 is a protein made by T-helper cells when they are stimulated by an infection. IL-2 is an immune modulator that strongly stimulates T-cell ($CD4^+$-cell) production.

4. C: Responsible for mucosal immunity

IgA accounts for approximately 15–20% of serum immunoglobulin (Ig) in secretions, saliva, tears, colostrum and bronchial/intestinal/gastrointestinal tract secretions. Serum IgA is largely monomeric but in secretions it exists as secretory IgA. A dimer of two IgA (IgA1 or IgA2) molecules bound by a J chain and attached to a molecule is known as the secretory piece. This piece is produced by the mucosa and facilitates the transport of secretory IgA (sIgA) into external secretions, which represents the first line of mucosal defence against bacteria and viruses. Production is stimulated by bacteria and viruses, which are removed by sIgA and phagocytosis.

5. A: TGF-β

The most important determinant of scarring in glomerulonephritis is believed to be proteinuria, which leads to activation of tubular epithelial cells and production of immune mediators including TGF-β. This leads to activation of interstitial cells and subsequent development of fibrosis and renal scarring.

6. A: Wegener's granulomatosis

Cytoplasmic anti-neutrophil cytoplasmic antibodies (c-ANCAs) are directed against constituents of the cytoplasm of neutrophils; c-ANCA is found in Wegener's granulomatosis where it is highly sensitive (90% of patients) and specific. Less commonly it is found in microscopic polyangiitis, whereas perinuclear ANCA (p-ANCA) is also found in microscopic polyangiitis, and more widely in connective tissue disorders and other vasculitides.

Essential Revision Notes for MRCP, 2nd edn, p 327

7. D: Sarcoidosis

Type IV hypersensitivity reactions are cell-mediated or delayed-type hypersensitivity, typified by the tuberculin reaction or graft-versus-host disease. In contrast, type I reactions are anaphylactic; type II reactions represent antibody-dependent cytotoxicity (eg Goodpasture syndrome), type III reactions represent immune complex-mediated (eg aspergillosis) ones and type V reactions are stimulatory (eg Graves' disease).

Essential Revision Notes for MRCP, 2nd edn, p 321

8. E: Anti-Ro

Neonatal complications of SLE can occur through transplacental transfer of autoantibodies, particularly anti-Ro. This can produce a transient photosensitive rash, complete heart block or thrombocytopenia.

Essential Revision Notes for MRCP, 2nd edn, p 707

9. E: Anti-mitochondrial antibodies

Anti-mitochondrial antibodies are present in 95% of individuals with primary biliary cirrhosis; 90% of patients are women.

Essential Revision Notes for MRCP, 2nd edn, p 223

10. D: BCG

BCG is a live attenuated vaccine and therefore should be avoided in immunocompromised individuals. In contrast, tetanus, varicella and diphtheria vaccines are preformed antibodies and hepatitis B is a subunit vaccine.

Essential Revision Notes for MRCP, 2nd edn, p 332

11. A: SCL-70

SCL-70 antibodies have low sensitivity but high specificity for systemic sclerosis, a connective tissue disorder characterised by thickening and fibrosis of the skin (scleroderma) plus involvement of internal organs.

Essential Revision Notes for MRCP, 2nd edn, p 710

12. E: Anti-acetylcholine receptor antibodies

This clinical history is typical of myasthenia gravis, the most common primary disorder of neuromuscular transmission. In this disorder, anti-acetylcholine receptor antibodies attack the post-synaptic acetylcholine receptors at the neuromuscular junction, inhibiting normal neuromuscular transmission.

Essential Revision Notes for MRCP, 2nd edn, p 584

13. D: TSH

Graves' disease is an example of a type V hypersensitivity reaction (*see* Question 7) and is a common cause of thyrotoxicosis. Anti-TSH antibodies are produced, which are stimulatory at the TSH receptor, leading to thyrotoxicosis.

Essential Revision Notes for MRCP, 2nd edn, p 137

14. B: Type II

Type II hypersensitivity reactions are mediated by antibody-dependent cytotoxicity. Examples include transfusion reactions and rhesus incompatibility, immune thrombocytopenia and Goodpasture syndrome

Essential Revision Notes for MRCP, 2nd edn, p 321

15. A: Yellow fever

Yellow fever vaccine is a live attenuated vaccine and should not therefore be given to immunocompromised patients. *See* Question 10.

Essential Revision Notes for MRCP, 2nd edn, p 332

16. E: Mouse B lymphocytes

Monoclonal antibody production occurs from mouse B-cell precursors (which mount a polyclonal immune response to an injected antigen); they are harvested and fused en masse to a specialised myeloma cell line. These immortal cell lines or hybridomas can then be screened to select for the monoclonal antibody of interest.

Essential Revision Notes for MRCP, 2nd edn, p 432

17. B: IgE

Immediate-type hypersensitivity represents an anaphylactic reaction where antigen combines with IgE on mast cells and basophils, leading to the release of vasoactive substances.

Essential Revision Notes for MRCP, 2nd edn, p 321

18. D: IgA

The classic pathway of complement activation is activated by antigen–antibody complexes containing IgM or IgG, whereas the alternative pathway is initiated by polysaccharides in the cell wall of Gram-negative bacteria as well as weakly by IgA.

Essential Revision Notes for MRCP, 2nd edn, p 311

19. C: Mast cells

Mast cells are a form of tissue-bound leucocytes and are not normally found in circulating blood. Basophils are a related but distinct form of cell that circulates. All the other cell types are predominantly found in the circulation.

Essential Revision Notes for MRCP, 2nd edn, p 317

20. B: B cells

Chronic lymphocytic leukaemia is the commonest of the lymphoproliferative disorders and is characterised by an excessive number of circulating B lymphocytes, together with bone marrow involvement, a variable degree of lymph node and splenic involvement, hypogammaglobulinaemia and haemolysis.

21. A: HLA-DR

HLA antigens are coded by genes on chromosome 6. For renal transplantation, HLA-DR and HLA-B matching have the strongest influence on graft survival for unknown reasons. Matching for HLA-A and HLA-C also improves graft survival.

Essential Revision Notes for MRCP, 2nd edn, p 492

22. A: T cells

Neutrophils are the commonest of the circulating white cells, making up about 60% of the circulating leucocytes. Lymphocytes are the second commonest group (~25%) and T cells make up the largest group. Monocytes, eosinophils and basophils each make up less than 10% of the circulating white blood cells. Mast cells are tissue bound and usually do not circulate in the blood stream.

23. E: Trastuzumab

Trastuzumab is a monoclonal antibody used in the treatment of HER2-positive breast cancer. It is thought to bind to HER2-receptor sites over-expressed in a proportion of breast cancers, preventing cellular growth through interruption of receptor function.

24. B: HIV

This is a typical clinical presentation for progressive multifocal leucoencephalopathy (PML), which is associated with the presence of the JC virus and with immunodeficiency. Pathologically, PML consists of multiple foci of demyelination that vary in size.

25. D: *Mycoplasma pneumoniae*

Elevated cold agglutinin titres are found in about half of patients with mycoplasma pneumonia. Other atypical pneumonias may induce low titres of cold agglutinins. The cold agglutinin is an antibody that will react with antigens on red blood cell glycoproteins, and the antibody is generated in response to a protein produced by mycoplasma that helps it attach to receptors on the respiratory epithelium.

26. A: *Staphylococcus aureus*

Disorders of neutrophil function are relatively uncommon and associated with low-grade chronic bacterial or fungal infections, most frequently with catalase-negative organisms such as *Staphylococcus aureus* and *Aspergillus* spp.

27. B: T-cell malignancy

Sézary syndrome is a cutaneous T-cell lymphoma associated with erythroderma, generalised lymphadenopathy and hepatosplenomegaly. Histologically it is characterised by Sézary cells that are $CD4^{+}$ T lymphocytes with an unusual convoluted morphology.

28. B: CD4

CD4 is a cell surface glycoprotein that is present on T-helper cells and monocytes. It recognises major histocompatibility complex (MHC) class II antigens on antigen-presenting cells. Interactions with CD4 and a co-receptor are usually essential for HIV to enter cells efficiently.

29. D: *Borrelia recurrentis*

Periodic variation in the antigens exposed by bacteria is one way to evade immune defences. Antigenic variation usually results from site-specific inversions, gene conversions or gene rearrangements in the DNA of the micro-organisms. *Borrelia recurrentis* is a spirochaete that causes the human disease relapsing fever, in which recurrent attacks are mediated by antigenically distinct mutants. *Neisseria gonorrhoeae* is another example of a bacterium that can undergo antigenic variation, changing fimbrial antigens during the course of an infection.

30. C: Langerhans' cells

Langerhans cells are dendritic cells located in the epidermis, and are part of the mononuclear phagocytic system that processes and presents foreign antigens to the immune system. Abnormal proliferation of Langerhans cells can occur in histiocytosis X.

31. C: Activation of NF-κB transcription factor

TNF-α is a pro-inflammatory cytokine with a wide range of effects, and is produced by macrophages, eosinophils and NK cells. NFκB is a nuclear transcription factor that is activated by TNF-α and plays an important role in the inflammatory process by inducing transcription of proinflammatory cytokines, chemokines, Cox-2 and adhesion molecules.

Essential Revision Notes for MRCP, 2nd edn, p 324

32. B: Mixed cryoglobulinaemia

Rheumatoid factor (RF) is an IgM antibody directed against the Fc portion of IgG. It is present in about 80% of patients with rheumatoid arthritis, and is also commonly positive in cryoglobulinaemia (where it may be very high in titre) or Sjögren syndrome.

Essential Revision Notes for MRCP, 2nd edn, p 695

33. D: Type IV

Graft-versus-host disease is an example of cell-mediated or delayed-type hypersensitivity (type IV). Presentation of antigen to sensitised memory T cells leads to T-cell activation and release of lymphokines. Other examples of type IV hypersensitivity reactions include contact dermatitis and the tuberculin reaction.

Essential Revision Notes for MRCP, 2nd edn, p 321

34. D: MHC class II interaction

CD4 is a glycoprotein found on the surface of T lymphocytes, monocytes, macrophages and dendritic cells. It is the major marker of T-helper cells, and binds to MHC class II molecules on antigen-presenting cells, thus enabling the recognition of specific antigens presented in association with the MHC molecules. CD4 is also the major receptor for the binding of HIV.

35. E: C5

Opportunistic bacterial infections, such as meningococcal infection and gonorrhoea, occur because of defects in the lytic complement pathway (C5–C9).

36. C: Renal biopsy

This clinical presentation is consistent with Goodpasture syndrome, which is characterised by the presence of circulating antibodies to the glomerular basement membrane. Specific biopsy changes are seen in this syndrome, with IgG deposited on the glomerular basement membrane in a linear fashion.

Essential Revision Notes for MRCP, 2nd edn, p 504

37. D: Takayasu's arteritis

Vasculitides are classified according to the size of the blood vessels commonly involved and/or the pattern of organ involvement. Kawasaki's disease and polyartertitis nodosa are non-granulomatous vasculitides of medium or small vessels, Wegener's granulomatosis is a granulomatous vasculitis of medium-sized vessels and cryoglobulinaemia affects small vessels. Takayasu's arteritis and giant cell arteritis, in contrast, principally affect large vessels.

Essential Revision Notes for MRCP, 2nd edn, p 714

38. A: Langerhans' cells

Antigen-presenting cells are specialised cells that process and 'present' antigen on their cell surface bound to MHC class II molecules. This allows T-cell receptors to recognise and bind to the antigen. Macrophages, follicular dendritic cells and Langerhans' cells are examples of antigen-presenting cells, the last being specific to the skin.

39. D: Limited scleroderma

Extractable nuclear antigens (Ro, La, Sm, RNP, Jo-1, Sc170, centromere) are specific nuclear antigens and so they are associated with a positive ANA. Anti-centromere antibodies are specifically associated with the CREST syndrome (limited scleroderma consisting of **c**alcinosis, **R**aynaud syndrome, o**e**sophageal dysmotility, **s**clerodactyly and **t**elangiectasia). Anti-Ro would be seen in Sjögren syndrome and anti-La in primary Sjögren syndrome; anti-RNP would be seen in mixed connective tissue disease.

Essential Revision Notes for MRCP, 2nd edn, pp 326, 711

40. B: Antibodies to dsDNA

High titres of anti-dsDNA are specific for SLE, and overall anti-dsDNA is seen in about 80% of patients with SLE. Some specific antibodies to extractable nuclear antigens are specific for SLE (eg anti-Sm very specific, conferring a high risk of renal lupus), but overall anti-ENAs are not specific and not seen in many other immunological disorders.

Essential Revision Notes for MRCP, 2nd edn, p 327

41. A: Cardiac fibrosis

Clinical features of Sjögren syndrome include dry membranes from atrophy of exocrine glands, arthritis, Raynaud's phenomenon, lymphadenopathy and parotid swelling, vasculitis, neuropathies, renal tubular acidosis and pancreatitis.

Essential Revision Notes for MRCP, 2nd edn, p 712

42. B: Ig light chains

Defective malignant plasma cells in myeloma cannot make a complete Ig molecule and are able to make only light chains. These are small enough to be filtered at the glomerulus and appear as Bence Jones proteinuria. By obstructing renal tubular function they can also contribute to the renal failure seen in myeloma.

Essential Revision Notes for MRCP, 2nd edn, p 290

43. E: Direct Coombs' test

The direct Coomb's test (direct antiglobulin test) is used to detect C3 or IgG bound to the surface of a red cell. In patients with evidence of haemolysis, this test is useful in determining whether there is an immunological aetiology. Spherocytes reflect either hereditary spherocytosis or an immunologically mediated haemolytic process. The probable clinical diagnosis here will be an autoimmune haemolytic anaemia, which would be best supported by a positive direct Coombs' test.

44. A: Absence of HLA-B27

Ankylosing spondylitis is an inflammatory disease of unknown cause characterised by inflammation of multiple joints, often leading to bony ankylosis. HLA-B27 has a sensitivity of approximately 95% for ankylosing spondylitis, although there is limited specificity as a result of the prevalence of HLA-B27 in the general population. Consequently although the presence of HLA-B27 does not particularly help in the diagnosis, its absence would be inconsistent with a diagnosis of ankylosing spondylitis.

Essential Revision Notes for MRCP, 2nd edn, p 704

45. A: Polyclonal origin

Myasthenia gravis is an autoimmune disorder of neuromuscular transmission that is caused by antibodies directed against the acetylcholine receptor. This is a polyclonal IgG antibody present in around 90–95% of patients which blocks neuromuscular transmission in a variety of ways: not only receptor blockade but also complement-mediated destruction of acetylcholine receptors.

Essential Revision Notes for MRCP, 2nd edn, p 584

46. B: High RF titre

Poor prognostic factors in rheumatoid arthritis include male sex, positive family history, age, high RF titre, evidence of extra-articular features or erosive disease.

47. D: Low levels of paraprotein

It is important to differentiate benign paraproteinaemia, or monoclonal gammopathy of uncertain significance (MGUS), from myeloma. About 10% of patients with MGUS develop myeloma within 5 years. A high or rising level of paraprotein, renal or bone involvement, or depressed levels of other immunoglobins are all more consistent with a diagnosis of myeloma.

Essential Revision Notes for MRCP, 2nd edn, p 291

48. B: c-ANCA

Anti-neutrophil cytoplasmic antibody, specifically c-ANCA with PR3 specificity, is the most specific autoantibody for Wegener's granulomatosis and is found in 90% of patients; p-ANCAs are found in perhaps 25%. Anti-Ro antibodies are found in Sjögren syndrome and some cases of SLE.

Essential Revision Notes for MRCP, 2nd edn, p 327

Chapter 7

STATISTICS, EPIDEMIOLOGY AND EVIDENCE-BASED MEDICINE

Questions

---

1. A new test for autism has recently been discovered. What term describes the proportion of patients with clinically confirmed autism who will be identified by the test?

☐ A Sensitivity

☐ B Specificity

☐ C Positive predictive value

☐ D Accuracy

☐ E Negative predictive value

2. A new diagnostic test for myocardial infarction (MI) is introduced. Which parameter will indicate the proportion of patients without an MI in whom the test will be negative?

☐ A Accuracy

☐ B Negative predictive value

☐ C Positive predictive value

☐ D Sensitivity

☐ E Specificity

3. The percentage of patients experiencing drug side effects is to be compared between two differently treated groups. What is the most appropriate statistical test?

- ☐ A Multiple linear regression
- ☐ B χ^2 (chi-squared) test
- ☐ C Mann–Whitney U test
- ☐ D Spearman's correlation coefficient
- ☐ E Wilcoxon's test

4. A new test for Alzheimer's disease has 80% sensitivity and 90% specificity. If, on average, 1 in 16 new patients presenting to a memory clinic has Alzheimer's disease, what are the odds that a patient testing positive on the new test actually has Alzheimer's disease?

- ☐ A 9 in 10
- ☐ B 4 in 5
- ☐ C 1 in 16
- ☐ D 1 in 13
- ☐ E 1 in 2

5. Which one of the following statements correctly describes the standard deviation of a group under observation?

- ☐ A It is the square of the variance of the group
- ☐ B It is a measure of the spread of the observations
- ☐ C It is valid only if the observations have a normal (gaussian) distribution
- ☐ D It is numerically lower than the standard error of the mean for the group
- ☐ E It is always larger than the mean of the observations

6. A new medication reduces the death rate from a disease from 50% to 30%. What is the number needed to treat to prevent one death?

- ☐ A 20
- ☐ B 50
- ☐ C 5
- ☐ D 10
- ☐ E 1

7. What is the power of a study?

- ☐ A Probability of correctly rejecting the null hypothesis
- ☐ B Probability of accepting the null hypothesis
- ☐ C Likelihood of a significant finding
- ☐ D The number of samples required for a positive finding
- ☐ E Likelihood of obtaining an answer

8. Which one of the following parameters concerning a screening test relates to the proportion of people without the disease correctly identified by the test?

- ☐ A Sensitivity
- ☐ B Specificity
- ☐ C Probability
- ☐ D Power
- ☐ E Positive predictive value

Answers on pages 187–206

9. To test the efficacy of a new drug versus placebo, a double-blind, randomised controlled trial is proposed. What is the best reason for using randomisation?

- ☐ A Prevents patients knowing which medication they are taking
- ☐ B Prevents physicians knowing which medication the patient is taking
- ☐ C Ensures that equal numbers of patients are recruited to each group
- ☐ D Ensures that the findings are statistically significant
- ☐ E Ensures that the two groups have similar characteristics at trial entry

10. A pharmaceutical company wants to assess rare adverse effects that are thought to occur in less than 1% of patients taking a new antihypertensive drug. What type of study is most appropriate for assessing these effects?

- ☐ A Phase I
- ☐ B Phase II
- ☐ C Phase III
- ☐ D Phase IV
- ☐ E Phase V

11. The blood pressure of a sample of 100 randomly selected individuals is measured. Which term describes how closely the mean blood pressure from this sample approximates the mean blood pressure in the general population?

- ☐ A Standard error
- ☐ B Standard deviation
- ☐ C 95% confidence interval
- ☐ D Mode
- ☐ E Median

12. Which one of the following is a parametric statistical test?

- ☐ A Mann–Whitney U test
- ☐ B Spearman's rank correlation
- ☐ C χ^2 test
- ☐ D Student's *t*-test
- ☐ E Sign test

13. In a clinical trial of a new treatment, under what situation is a type II error most likely to occur?

- ☐ A If the sample size is small
- ☐ B If the effect size is large
- ☐ C If multiple statistical tests are used
- ☐ D If the data are normally distributed
- ☐ E If the hypothesis under consideration is false

Answers on pages 187–206

14. A new screening test for colorectal cancer has a sensitivity of 90% and a specificity of 50%. Which one of the following statements about this test is correct?

- ☐ A Half those who do not have colorectal cancer will test positive
- ☐ B Half those who do have colorectal cancer will test positive
- ☐ C Of every 10 individuals who test positive, one will have the disease
- ☐ D Of every 10 individuals who test positive, nine will have the disease
- ☐ E It will be useful only in populations with a high incidence of colorectal cancer

15. Which one of the following statements is correct if a characteristic is normally distributed in a population?

- ☐ A Standard deviation will be equal to the variance
- ☐ B The median and the mean must differ
- ☐ C The mean and the mode will differ
- ☐ D Most of the population are normal
- ☐ E There will be equal numbers of individuals above and below the mean

16. Recall bias is most likely to be a problem in which of the following types of study?

- ☐ A Meta-analyses
- ☐ B Case–control studies
- ☐ C Cohort studies
- ☐ D Randomised controlled trials
- ☐ E Cross-over trials

17. In a clinical trial of a new treatment, under what situation is a type I error most likely to occur?

- ☐ A If the sample size is small
- ☐ B If the effect size is large
- ☐ C If multiple statistical tests are used
- ☐ D If the data are normally distributed
- ☐ E If the hypothesis under consideration is false

18. Which statement best describes the difference between the mean and the median value of the weights of a large number of patients attending a diabetic clinic?

- ☐ A It is identical to the standard deviation
- ☐ B It is smaller for positively skewed distributions
- ☐ C It represents the standard error
- ☐ D It is larger for positively skewed distributions
- ☐ E It is proportional to the number of patients measured

19. In a given population, which one of the following rates best reflects a change in the balance of aetiological factors of a particular disease?

- ☐ A Incidence
- ☐ B Point prevalence
- ☐ C Period prevalence
- ☐ D Five-year mortality rate
- ☐ E Standardised mortality ratio

Answers on pages 187–206

20. Which one of the following pieces of information is most likely to be obtained from post-marketing surveillance of 10 000 patients given a new drug?

- ☐ A Adverse events profile
- ☐ B Cost–benefit analysis
- ☐ C Cost-effectiveness
- ☐ D Comparative therapeutic efficacy
- ☐ E Drug potency

21. A screening programme for breast cancer results in a high number of cancers occurring in the interval between screening appointments. What is the most likely cause for this?

- ☐ A Screening test is too sensitive
- ☐ B Screening test has too low a positive predictive value
- ☐ C Screening test is too specific
- ☐ D Screening interval is too long
- ☐ E Screening interval is too short

22. Which one of the following terms best describes a simple linear regression?

- ☐ A Line going through the origin
- ☐ B Line with a positive slope
- ☐ C Curve describing the relationship between two variables
- ☐ D Line with a negative slope
- ☐ E Line intersecting the mean of two variables

23. Which one of the following factors is most important for taking into account when calculating how many patients should be recruited into a trial of a new drug therapy?

- ☐ A Cost of the drug
- ☐ B Prevalence of side effects
- ☐ C Prevalence of disease
- ☐ D Likely size of the treatment effect
- ☐ E Likelihood of drug interactions

24. A trial of a new drug for stroke finds that it reduces the mortality rate from 10% to 4%. What is the absolute risk reduction?

- ☐ A 2.5%
- ☐ B 4%
- ☐ C 6%
- ☐ D 10%
- ☐ E 250%

25. A trial of a new drug after stroke finds that it reduces the mortality rate from 10% to 4%. How many patients need to be treated with this drug to prevent one death?

- ☐ A 4
- ☐ B 10
- ☐ C 17
- ☐ D 40
- ☐ E 137

Answers on pages 187–206

26. Which one of the following is a measure of absolute risk?

- ☐ A Incidence rate ratio
- ☐ B Rate difference
- ☐ C Odds ratio
- ☐ D Hazard ratio
- ☐ E Risk ratio

27. The peak expiratory flow rate (PEFR) measurements of a group of medical students are normally distributed with a mean of 600 l/min and standard deviation 50 l/min. Which one of the following statements is most likely to be correct?

- ☐ A All PEFR measurements will be below 700 l/min
- ☐ B About 67% of the medical students will have PEFR between 500 and 700 l/min
- ☐ C About 50% of the medical students will have PEFR between 500 and 700 l/min
- ☐ D About 50% of the medical students will have a PEFR above 600 l/min
- ☐ E About 10% of the medical students will have a PEFR below 500 l/min

28. Which one of the following statements about a prospective epidemiological study of children at risk of developing a disease is correct?

- ☐ A It can determine disease prevalence
- ☐ B It can determine disease incidence
- ☐ C It is best suited to studying rare diseases
- ☐ D It will always be biased
- ☐ E It cannot determine risk factors for the disease

29. The effect of a new oral hypoglycaemic drug on blood glucose levels is measured in 20 healthy volunteers. Which statistical test will be most appropriate for determining whether the drug has a significant effect?

- ☐ A Mann–Whitney U test
- ☐ B Paired *t*-test
- ☐ C Multiple linear regression
- ☐ D Cross-correlation coefficient
- ☐ E χ^2 test

30. An asymptomatic individual enquires about screening for intracranial aneurysms. What action is the most appropriate?

- ☐ A Contrast-enhanced computed tomography (CT)
- ☐ B Magnetic resonance angiography (MRA)
- ☐ C No further action
- ☐ D Plain skull X-ray
- ☐ E Cerebral angiogram

31. A correlation coefficient between two variables is most likely to indicate which one of the following?

- ☐ A How closely the pairs of values lie to a straight line
- ☐ B Whether the pairs of values are consistently greater than zero
- ☐ C Increases in one variable are always accompanied by increases in the other
- ☐ D Whether the relationship between the two variables is statistically significant
- ☐ E Whether one variable is significantly greater than the other

32. Which one of the following is most likely to affect the statistical power of a randomised controlled trial?

- ☐ A Effect size
- ☐ B Quality of randomisation
- ☐ C Investigator blinding
- ☐ D Quality of subgroup analyses
- ☐ E Type of drug

33. Which one of the following statistical tests is most likely to be appropriate for an initial comparison of the mean level of blood pressure in three different patient groups?

- ☐ A Multidimensional scaling
- ☐ B Cluster analysis
- ☐ C Paired *t*-test
- ☐ D Analysis of variance
- ☐ E Independent component analysis

34. Which one of the following is most likely to be affected by selection bias?

- ☐ A Double-blind study
- ☐ B Cluster of randomised controlled trials
- ☐ C Randomised controlled trial
- ☐ D Cohort study
- ☐ E Phase III trial

35. Which one of the following types of bias is a randomised controlled trial most likely to minimise?

- ☐ A Recall
- ☐ B Selection
- ☐ C Criterion
- ☐ D Analysis
- ☐ E Media

36. Which one of the following statistical tests is best for comparing the cholesterol levels of a group of patients before and after lipid-lowering therapy?

- ☐ A χ^2 test
- ☐ B Paired *t*-test
- ☐ C Multiple linear regression
- ☐ D Cross-correlation
- ☐ E Kolmogorov–Smirnov test

37. Which one of the following is a property of the normal distribution?

- ☐ A All observations are within 1 SD of the mean
- ☐ B The mean is greater than the mode
- ☐ C All observations are within 2 SD of the mean
- ☐ D The mean, median and mode coincide
- ☐ E It is not significantly different from zero

38. Under which one of the following conditions will a *t*-test that compares two independent distributions be most likely to be valid?

- ☐ A Number of samples in each distribution small
- ☐ B Identical number of samples in each distribution
- ☐ C Both distributions normally distributed
- ☐ D Equal variance of the two distributions
- ☐ E Equal means of two distributions

39. After a trial of a new drug treatment aimed at reducing mortality as a result of stroke in 1000 patients, the NNT is calculated to be 50. What is the best interpretation of these findings?

- ☐ A 50 lives will be saved by treating 1000 patients
- ☐ B 20 lives will be saved by treating 1000 patients
- ☐ C 20 lives will be saved by treating 50 patients
- ☐ D 1 life will be saved by treating 1000 patients
- ☐ E 1 life will be saved by treating 50 patients

40. It is hypothesised that many men diagnosed as having colorectal cancer also suffer high rates of divorce. What type of study design would be best to test this hypothesis?

- ☐ A Prospective cohort study
- ☐ B Prospective, randomised controlled trial
- ☐ C Phase II trial
- ☐ D Retrospective case–control study
- ☐ E Prospective observational study

41. The standard deviation of the systolic blood pressure in a sample of 100 patients is 15.5 mmHg. What is the standard error of the mean of this measurement?

- ☐ A 155 mmHg
- ☐ B 15.5 mmHg
- ☐ C 1.55 mmHg
- ☐ D 0.155 mmHg
- ☐ E None of these

42. Which one of the following types of graph is useful for exploring publication bias?

- ☐ A Polar plot
- ☐ B Frequency plot
- ☐ C Regression plot
- ☐ D Scatter plot
- ☐ E Funnel plot

43. The correlation coefficient between the weight of a group of patients and their CD4 count is found to be 0.3. Which one of the following statements is most likely to be correct?

- ☐ A There is no significant relationship between weight and CD4 count
- ☐ B Patients with higher CD4 counts tend to have lower weights
- ☐ C Patients with higher CD4 counts tend to have higher weights
- ☐ D The relationship between CD4 count and weight is non-linear
- ☐ E The relationship between CD4 count and weight is strong

44. Which one of the following statements is most likely to be correct concerning a positively skewed distribution?

- ☐ A Mean less than median
- ☐ B Mean greater than mode
- ☐ C Mode greater than median
- ☐ D Mode greater than mean
- ☐ E Median greater than mean

45. The systolic blood pressure of a large number of patients with rheumatoid arthritis is normally distributed and has a mean of 130 mmHg, with a standard deviation of 12 mmHg. Approximately what proportion of observations will fall within 2 SD of the mean?

- ☐ A 50%
- ☐ B 67%
- ☐ C 75%
- ☐ D 95%
- ☐ E 100%

46. A new blood test to diagnose pulmonary embolism (PE) is performed on 100 patients with suspected PE. Of 20 people eventually diagnosed with PE, 15 tested positive with the blood test. In addition, five people without PE tested positive with the blood test. What is the sensitivity and specificity of this test?

- ☐ A Sensitivity 94%, specificity 75%
- ☐ B Sensitivity 75%, specificity 75%
- ☐ C Sensitivity 94%, specificity 94%
- ☐ D Sensitivity 20%, specificity 95%
- ☐ E Sensitivity 75%, specificity 94%

47. A 26-year-old presents with his first unprovoked grand-mal seizure. What period of time will his UK driving licence be suspended for?

- ☐ A Not until diagnosis of epilepsy reached
- ☐ B One month
- ☐ C Six months
- ☐ D One year
- ☐ E Five years

48. Which one of the following diseases is not notifiable in the UK?

- ☐ A Chlamydia infection
- ☐ B Tetanus
- ☐ C Diphtheria
- ☐ D Anthrax
- ☐ E Tuberculosis (TB)

49. What is the leading cause of cancer death in women in the UK?

- ☐ A Breast cancer
- ☐ B Ovarian cancer
- ☐ C Cervical cancer
- ☐ D Colorectal cancer
- ☐ E Brain cancer

50. In a clinical trial of a new vaccine, under what situation is a type I error most likely to occur?

- ☐ A If the data are not normally distributed
- ☐ B If only a small number of individuals are studied
- ☐ C If the hypothesis under consideration is false
- ☐ D If multiple statistical tests are used
- ☐ E If the effect size is large

51. A screening questionnaire is developed for use in suspected Alzheimer's disease. Which one of the following measures are likely to be identical whether the test is used in primary care or hospital practice?

- ☐ A Positive predictive value
- ☐ B Sensitivity
- ☐ C Negative predictive value
- ☐ D Prevalence
- ☐ E Incidence

52. Which one of the following is least likely to undermine the conclusions of a meta-analysis?

- ☐ A Symmetrical funnel plot
- ☐ B Selection bias
- ☐ C Publication bias
- ☐ D Statistical heterogeneity
- ☐ E Clinical heterogeneity

53. In a randomised controlled trial testing the effect of a drug treatment on recurrent MI, which one of the following measures are independent of the expected rate of recurrent infarction?

- ☐ A Overall outcome
- ☐ B NNT
- ☐ C Relative risk reduction
- ☐ D Absolute risk reduction
- ☐ E Study power

54. The forced expiratory volume in 1 s (FEV_1) is measured in 100 students, yielding a mean value of 4.5 l with a standard deviation of 0.5 l. Assuming that these values are normally distributed, what is the standard error of the mean?

- ☐ A 5
- ☐ B 1
- ☐ C 0.5
- ☐ D 0.05
- ☐ E 0.01

55. The FEV_1 is measured in 100 students, yielding a mean value of 4.5 l with a standard deviation of 0.5 l. Assuming that these values are normally distributed, what is the approximate 95% confidence interval for the population mean FEV_1?

- ☐ A 4.4–4.6 l
- ☐ B 4.0–5.0 l
- ☐ C 3.5–5.5 l
- ☐ D 4.2–4.8 l
- ☐ E Impossible to calculate

56. Which one of the following conditions is most likely to support a causal association of an aetiological factor with a disease?

- ☐ A The factor is found among all patients with the disease
- ☐ B Exposure to the factor occurs after diagnosis with the disease
- ☐ C The factor is found more frequently among those with the disease versus those without
- ☐ D The factor is not found among any patients who do not have the disease
- ☐ E Elimination of the factor does not alter the likelihood of disease

57. Which one of the following factors is most likely to affect the prevalence of a disease in a community?

- ☐ A Clinical significance
- ☐ B Duration
- ☐ C Relative risk
- ☐ D Positive predictive value
- ☐ E Infectivity

58. In a randomised controlled trial of a new drug treatment for incontinence, which one of the following statements best describes a type II error?

- ☐ A The α error
- ☐ B Risk of a false-positive result
- ☐ C Risk of a false-negative result
- ☐ D Risk of failing to recruit enough patients
- ☐ E The β error

59. A trial of a new treatment for pancreatic cancer finds that it reduces the mortality rate from 50% to 35%. What is the relative risk reduction for this treatment?

- ☐ A 0.5
- ☐ B 0.35
- ☐ C 0.3
- ☐ D 0.15
- ☐ E 0.1

60. A new brain scan to diagnose depression is performed on 200 patients with suspected depression. Of 20 people eventually diagnosed with depression, 5 tested positive with the brain scan. In addition, 20 people without depression tested positive with the brain scan. What is the sensitivity and specificity of this test?

- ☐ A Sensitivity 89%, specificity 89%
- ☐ B Sensitivity 10%, specificity 10%
- ☐ C Sensitivity 89%, specificity 25%
- ☐ D Sensitivity 25%, specificity 89%
- ☐ E Sensitivity 90%, specificity 90%

Answers on pages 187–206

STATISTICS, EPIDEMIOLOGY AND EVIDENCE-BASED MEDICINE

Answers

---

1. A: Sensitivity

The sensitivity of a test for a disease refers to how well that test correctly identifies people who have that disease – the probability that the test will produce a true positive result when used on a population with the disease (as compared to a reference or 'gold standard'). A test with high sensitivity will have few false negatives. The specificity of a test, on the other hand, is concerned with how well the test can correctly identify people who do not have the disease. A test with high specificity will have few false positives. The positive predictive value of a test is the probability that a person has the disease when a positive test result is observed. On the other hand, the negative predictive value of a test is the probability that a person does not have the disease when a negative test result is observed. Sensitivity and specificity are both measures of the accuracy of a diagnostic test.

2. E: Specificity

Sensitivity measures the proportion of patients with the disease who will test positive for the disease. Specificity measures the proportion of patients without the disease who will also test negative for the disease.

3. B: χ^2 test

The χ^2 test can be used to compare categorical measures, such as the percentage experiencing side effects in each of these two groups.

4. E: 1 in 2

The positive likelihood ratio for a test represents by how much to increase the probability of some disease being present if the test is positive. It is defined as the ratio of the probability of an individual *with* the condition having a positive test to the probability of an individual *without* the condition having a positive test, ie the sensitivity divided by (1 – specificity). In this case, the positive likelihood ratio is therefore 0.8/(1 – 0.9) = 8. After a positive test, the post-test odds of the disease being present are the pre-test odds multiplied by the likelihood ratio, ie (1/16) x 8 or 1 in 2.

5. B: It is a measure of the spread of the observations

The standard deviation (SD) is the square root of the variance and is the most commonly used measure of spread of a distribution. In a normal distribution, about 68% of the values are within 1 SD of the mean and about 95% of the values are within 2 SD of the mean. The standard error of the mean (SEM) will be numerically lower than the standard deviation (it is the standard deviation divided by the square root of the number of values).

6. C: 5

The number needed to treat (NNT) is the number of patients who need to be treated to prevent one additional bad outcome, eg if a drug has an NNT of 5, it means that five people have to be treated with the drug to prevent one additional bad outcome. The NNT is calculated as the inverse of the absolute risk reduction; here the absolute risk reduction is the difference between the untreated event rate (50 per 100) and the treated event rate (30 per 100), ie 20%. The NNT is therefore 5.

7. A: Probability of correctly rejecting the null hypothesis

The power of a study is the likelihood (normally expressed as a percentage) of correctly rejecting the null hypothesis when it is false.

8. B: Specificity

The sensitivity of a test for a disease refers to how well that test correctly identifies people who have that disease. *See* Questions 1 and 2.

9. E: Ensures that the two groups have similar characteristics at trial entry

Randomisation ensures that the demographic characteristics and expected outcomes of the two groups should be similar at trial entry. The double-blind nature of this trial ensures that neither patients nor their physicians are aware of which medication they are taking. The statistical significance of the findings has nothing to do with randomisation but instead reflects the power of the study to detect any differences that may exist.

10. D: Phase IV

Phase I trials are used to test a new drug or treatment in a small number of individuals for the first time to evaluate safety, determine safe dosage range and identify important side effects. In phase II trials, the drug or treatment is given to a larger group of people (about 100) to confirm efficacy and further investigate the side effects. Phase III trials are in larger groups of people (about 1000) to confirm effectiveness and monitor side effects. Phase IV trials involve post-launch safety surveillance of a new drug or treatment, so phase IV trials are the type of study most suitable for investigating a relatively rare side effect. Phase V trials are for new indications and repeat phases II and III.

11. A: Standard error

The standard deviation is a measure of variability. For a sample of blood pressure values, it is a measure of the variability of the population from which the sample was drawn. In contrast, the standard error is an estimate of the precision of the sample mean.

12. D: Student's *t*-test

Parametric statistical tests are used when the data are normally distributed. Pearson's correlation coefficient and Student's *t*-test are examples of parametric tests. Non-parametric tests are used when the data are not normally distributed, and are normally based on ranking the data.

Essential Revision Notes for MRCP, 2nd edn, p 735

13. A: If the sample size is small

A type II error is the mistaken acceptance of the null hypothesis (no difference between new treatment and control, in this case) when it is in fact false. This would be the case if the trial found no evidence of efficacy of the new treatment when it was in fact efficacious. A type II error is most likely to occur when the power of the study to detect such differences is small, eg if only a small number of patients are recruited, or if the effect size is very small. Repeated statistical testing is more likely to lead to a false-positive (type I error) finding.

Essential Revision Notes for MRCP, 2nd edn, p 734

14. A: Half those who do not have colorectal cancer will test positive

Sensitivity is the proportion of true positives (in this case, people who do have colorectal cancer) correctly identified by the test. Specificity is the proportion of true negatives (people who do not have colorectal cancer) correctly identified by the test. A specificity of 50% means that 50% of people who do not have colorectal cancer will test negative. As this means that the other 50% will test positive (falsely), Answer A is the best one.

Essential Revision Notes for MRCP, 2nd edn, pp 738–9

15. E: There will be equal numbers of individuals above and below the mean

Mean, median and mode will be equal for a normally distributed characteristic, which refers to the shape of the distribution rather than to whether the individuals are 'normal' or 'abnormal' for that characteristic. Standard deviation is the positive square root of variance. For a normal distribution, half the values will lie above the mean.

16. B: Case–control studies

Recall bias is most likely to occur when participants in a study are asked about their experience, risk factors or behaviour after they have been diagnosed with the disease under study, eg in a case–control study, patients diagnosed with a particular disorder may recall aspects of their personal histories differently from people who do not have the disease.

17. C: If multiple statistical tests are used

A type I error is a false-positive rejection of the null hypothesis when it is in fact true. False positives are not particularly likely to occur with small sample sizes (false negatives will be more common) or if the effect size is large. However, if multiple statistical tests are used without any correction for multiple comparisons this increases the chance of a false-positive test result.

18. B: It is smaller for positively skewed distributions

The mean and median are identical for normally distributed data, and are unrelated to the standard deviation, which is a measure of the variability in the measured characteristic. In a skewed distribution of values, the median is generally a better summary of the data and is smaller than the mean for positively skewed deviations (and greater than the mean for negatively skewed distributions).

19. A: Incidence

Changing aetiological factors are likely to result in a change in the likelihood of individuals in a given population developing that disease. The prevalence of a condition in a population at one point in time is the point prevalence, whereas the period prevalence measures the prevalence over a period of time (eg a year). The incidence of a disease is the number of new occurrences of that disease in a given population over a period of time. As individuals with a history of that disease are not included (only new diagnoses), the incidence will best reflect changing likelihood of developing the disease as a result of changes in aetiological factors. Changes in the likelihood of developing a disease will not be directly reflected in mortality rates or ratios for individuals who have that disease.

20. A: Adverse events profile

Post-launch surveillance is most likely to pick up relatively rare adverse events. By this stage therapeutic efficacy and drug potency will already have been addressed before the drug obtained a licence, plus appropriate cost–benefit analyses.

21. D: Screening interval is too long

The success of a screening programme for cancer depends not only on the earlier detection of cancers at screening but also on the low rates of interval cancers arising between screenings. An overly sensitive screening test would lead to over-diagnosis of cancer at screening, rather than interval cancers. The positive predictive value of the test refers to those who actually test positive and so is not directly relevant to interval cancers, and the specificity of the test refers to those without the disease. The best answer here is that the screening interval is too long, leading to interval cancers.

22. E: Line intersecting the mean of two variables

Linear regression is a mathematical procedure for estimating whether one variable can be accurately predicted from another using a simple linear equation, describing the relationship between the two variables in terms of a line of certain slope plus an intercept (offset) value. The line relating the two variables therefore does not have to go through the origin (if the intercept is non-zero), does not have to have a positive (or negative) slope and is a line (hence linear) rather than a curve. The line intersects the mean of each variable, making E the best answer.

Essential Revision Notes for MRCP, 2nd edn, p 738

23. D: Likely size of the treatment effect

In terms of determining the efficacy, the likely size of any treatment effect is the primary determinant for deciding how many patients need to be recruited. The cost of the drug, or its potential side effects and interactions, are ethically important, but do not directly enter into any power calculation.

24. C: 6%

The absolute risk reduction is a measure of the effects of a treatment that compares the probability of some type of outcome in the treatment groups with that in a control group. It is expressed as a simple difference in the proportion in each group with the given effects. In the current example, the absolute risk reduction is the difference in relative risk reduction in the drug group and control group.

25. C: 17

See answer to Question 6.

26. B: Rate difference

The two main measures of absolute risk are the rate difference (the difference between incidence rates for a disease in groups exposed to different conditions) and the risk difference (difference in average risks in groups exposed to different conditions).

Essential Revision Notes for MRCP, 2nd edn, p 161

27. D: About 50% of the medical students will have a PEFR above 600 l/min

The standard deviation is a statistical measure of variability about a mean. When the variable in question is normally distributed, two-thirds of the scores on this variable will be within 1 SD of the mean, and 95% of the scores within 2 SD of the mean. Thus A is incorrect (there will be some PEFR measurements > 700 l/min), B is incorrect (this would be correct for 550–650 l/min), and C and E are incorrect.

28. B: It can determine disease incidence

Incidence of a disease is the frequency of new occurrences over a defined time interval. A prospective study accumulates cases over time and so is able to determine disease incidence, but it will not be possible to establish disease prevalence. This is because prevalence is the ratio of the number of cases of a disease present in the population at a specified time and the number of individuals in the population at that specified time, and a prospective study is unable to determine either.

29. B: Paired *t*-test

A paired *t*-test allows a comparison of the means of two samples, when each observation in one sample is specifically matched with an observation in the other. Here, pre-/post-blood glucose levels are naturally matched, being from the same individuals, so a paired *t*-test will be most appropriate for comparing the values.

30. C: No further action

Screening of asymptomatic patients without any risk factors for intracranial aneurysm does not provide any benefits, probably as a result of the relatively low incidence of intracranial aneurysm coupled with their low rate of rupture and the complications associated with neurosurgical intervention in asymptomatic individuals. Screening of patients with a positive family history or risk factors is more controversial.

31. A: How closely the pairs of values lie to a straight line

The more closely points representing the relationship between two different variables lie to a straight line, the more closely the two are associated and the higher the probability that one of the variables can be accurately predicted given only the value of the other. It has nothing to do with whether the values are greater or less than zero, or with the form of the relationship (positive or negative) between the two variables, or whether the two ranges of variable values are significantly different.

Essential Revision Notes for MRCP, 2nd edn, p 736

32. A: Effect size

The power of a study is an estimate of its ability correctly to reject the null hypothesis (eg for a trial of a new drug, correctly to reject the null hypothesis of no difference with drug treatment if the drug is indeed efficacious). It will depend strongly on the effect size (if a drug produces a large effect, fewer participants and/or less follow-up will be necessary to reject the null hypothesis correctly). The quality of randomisation will also affect the overall power (by introducing bias) as will investigator blinding, but effect size is a better overall answer given its dominant effect.

33. D: Analysis of variance

The initial biological question here is whether there are any systematic differences in the mean blood pressure among the three different groups. Analysis of variance is a statistical procedure for evaluating the differences in the means of two or more groups of cases.

34. D: Cohort study

Selection bias is potential bias introduced into a study by selecting different types of people into treatment and comparison groups. These differences then confound interpretation of any differences caused by the treatment. The various forms of randomisation in randomised controlled trials (including phase III trials) are designed to counter this, although some selection bias may occur. Non-randomised observational studies such as cohort studies are therefore more susceptible to selection bias.

35. B: Selection

See Question and answer 34.

36. B: Paired *t*-test

See Question and answer 29.

37. D: The mean, median and mode coincide

A variable follows a normal distribution if it is continuous and its frequency distribution follows the characteristic, symmetrical, bell-shaped form in which all the values of mean, median and mode coincide. About two-thirds of observations are within 1 SD of the mean and 95% within 2 SD.

38. C: Both distributions normally distributed

The *t*-test is a statistical procedure that computes the probability that two samples are members of the same population. For two different distributions, it therefore estimates the likelihood that they in fact belong to the same underlying distribution (rather than represent two different distributions). It is a requirement of a *t*-test that the samples be normally distributed and so this is the best answer.

39. E: 1 life is saved by treating 50 patients

See Question 25. The number of patients in the trial is not relevant once the NNT has been calculated.

40. D: Retrospective case–control study

In a retrospective case–control study, cases with colorectal cancer are identified and matched with controls who do not have the disease. Rates of divorce can then be systematically compared between the two groups. Prospective trials (eg observational study) could also detect a causal relationship between these two factors, but are not the best answer because they would take considerably longer to determine (and in the case of randomised controlled trials will be unethical because it would not be appropriate to randomise patients to either divorce or no-divorce arms!).

41. C: 1.55 mmHg

The standard error of the mean is a measure of variability in a sample that quantifies how accurately the underlying population mean is known. The larger the sample size, the smaller the standard error of the mean (reflecting increasing certainty that we know the underlying population mean). Formally, the standard error is calculated as the standard deviation divided by the square root of the sample size (here, the square root of 100 because this number of patients has been studied).

42. E: Funnel plot

A funnel plot allows comparison of the results of a number of different studies on some condition or treatment. An estimate of effect size is plotted against a measure of study size. Points that deviate from a symmetrical funnel shape can indicate publication bias (the tendency for striking findings to be published even if spurious, and for studies with statistically non-significant findings to remain unpublished).

Essential Revision Notes for MRCP, 2nd edn, p 172

43. C: Patients with higher CD4 counts tend to have higher weights

The correlation coefficient describes the strength of association between two variables.

44. B: Mean greater than mode

A positively skewed distribution has a long 'tail' of high values, and so the median is lower than the mean, and the mode is even lower than the median.

Essential Revision Notes for MRCP, 2nd edn, p 730

45. D: 95%

For a normally distributed population of samples, about two-thirds of the values will lie within ±1 standard deviations from the mean, and approximately 95% of the observations within ±2 standard deviations from the mean.

Essential Revision Notes for MRCP, 2nd edn, p 731

46. E: Sensitivity 75%, specificity 94%

Sensitivity represents the proportion of patients with PE who are correctly diagnosed by the test – in this case 15 out of 20, ie 75%. The specificity represents the proportion of patients without PE correctly diagnosed by a negative test. In this case, 80 individuals did not have PE and 75 of them had a negative test so the specificity is 75/80 or 94%.

47. D: One year

After an unprovoked seizure, it is the law that UK citizens must notify the Driver and Vehicle Licensing Agency (DVLA). Normally the DVLA will require individuals to stop driving and surrender their licences until they have been completely seizure free for a year. Individuals (not doctors) must inform the DVLA regardless of whether they have been diagnosed with epilepsy (or any other condition) and regardless of whether they had a tonic–clonic or other type of seizure.

48. A: Chlamydia infection

Notifiable diseases in the UK are:
Acute encephalitis
Acute poliomyelitis
Anthrax
Cholera
Diphtheria
Dysentery
Food poisoning
Leprosy
Leptospirosis
Malaria
Measles
Meningitis
Meningococcal septicaemia
Mumps
Ophthalmia neonatorum
Paratyphoid fever
Plague
Rabies
Relapsing fever
Rubella
Scarlet fever
Smallpox
Tetanus
TB
Typhoid fever
Typhus fever
Viral haemorrhagic fever
Viral hepatitis
Whooping cough
Yellow fever

49. A: Breast cancer

Breast cancer is the most common cancer in the UK, with around 36 000 new cases diagnosed per annum in England, which is about one-third of all cancers in women. There are about 10 000 deaths per annum from breast cancer in England.

50. D: If multiple statistical tests are used

See answer to Question 13

51. B: Sensitivity

The sensitivity of the test will be identical because it refers to the proportion of patients with the disease correctly identified by the test. However, both incidence and prevalence of Alzheimer's disease (and many other diseases) will vary between primary and secondary care. Crucially, the positive (and negative) predictive value of tests depends not only on their sensitivity and specificity, but also on the prior probability of the disease being present (and thus on the prevalence and incidence statistics that will change between primary and secondary care).

52. A: Symmetrical funnel plot

Although a funnel plot can be very useful in assessing publication bias in meta-analyses (*see* Question 42), it does not on its own add much weight to evaluating the overall strength of the meta-analysis. Selection and publication bias (plus other forms of bias) can influence which studies are included in the meta-analysis and therefore potentially strongly undermine its conclusions. Similarly, clinical heterogeneity of the population under study and statistical heterogeneity of the findings can potentially strongly undermine any meta-analytical conclusions.

53. C: Relative risk reduction

The relative risk of an event (in this case, recurrent MI) comparing the treated and control groups will be independent of the exact expected event rate. This means that the relative risk measure from a trial can be directly applied to any group of patients, irrespective of their precise event rate. However, the absolute risk reduction and NNT will depend on the expected event rate.

54. D: 0.05

The standard error of the mean is a measure of how closely the mean of some sample of values approximates the general population mean for those values. It is calculated from the standard deviation by dividing by the square root of the number of observations. The standard error of the mean is therefore smaller for larger sample sizes, reflecting the increased precision of the sample estimate.

Essential Revision Notes for MRCP, 2nd edn, pp 731–2

55. A: 4.4–4.6 l

This is another way of enquiring about measures of how precisely the mean of a sample approximates the mean of an underlying (unobserved) set of samples, but here by enquiring about confidence intervals. The interval defined by the sample mean plus or minus two times the standard error of the mean is an approximate 95% confidence interval. As the standard error is 0.05, the 95% confidence interval will be in the range 4.5 ± 0.1 l. *See* Question 54.

Essential Revision Notes for MRCP, 2nd edn, p 732

56. C: The factor is found more frequently among those with the disease versus those without

The key point to appreciate is that the potentially causal aetiological factor must occur more frequently in patients with the disease compared with those without. This relative frequency is more important than the absolute frequency either in the diseased alone, or in those without the disease considered alone (for each of these values give no information about the relative frequency).

57. B: Duration

The prevalence of a disease is the ratio of the number of cases of a disease present in a particular population at a specified time to the overall number of individuals in that population. For a given disease, the prevalence therefore depends on both the incidence of the disease and the duration of time that individuals are affected.

58. C: Risk of a false-negative result

A type II or β error occurs when the null hypothesis is wrongly accepted (ie a false-negative finding). A type I or α error represents a false-positive finding, when the null hypothesis is wrongly rejected.

59. C: 0.3

The relative risk reduction describes how much risk is reduced in the treatment group compared with the control group. The difference in the event rates between the two groups is divided by the event rate in the control group to determine the relative risk reduction, expressed either as a fraction or as a percentage. Here, the reduction in events is (0.5 – 0.35) so the relative risk reduction is (0.5 – 0.35)/0.5 = 0.3 or 30%.

60. D: Sensitivity 25%, specificity 89%

Sensitivity represents the proportion of patients with depression who are correctly diagnosed by the test. In this case, this is 5 out of 20, ie 25%. The specificity represents the proportion of patients without depression correctly diagnosed by a negative test. In this case, 180 individuals did not have depression and 160 of them had a negative test so the specificity is 160/180 or 89%.

Index

Locators are given as chapter number.question number.